Shaking Hands with Alzheimer's Disease:
A Guide to Compassion for Caretakers
of People with Alzheimer's Disease

The Seven Steps of Compassionate Caregiving

Maria "Dr. Mo" Pertik, RN, PhD
and Zora de Bodisco

This book is dedicated to my mother, Elena Pertik, MD, and to my father, Thomas Zoltan Pertik, Wadim de Bodisco, and all those who care for Alzheimer's patients.

It is meant to be used by families, financial institutions, law enforcement, insurance companies, and care facilities.

The book presents options for intentionally creating compassion and making a difference in the quality of life for individuals with Alzheimer's disease.

Contents

ACKNOWLEDGMENTS

In my role as a nurse, therapist, educator, and caretaker, my hands have touched those of so many people living with Alzheimer's disease that I have lost count of the number. When I think of those many people, I clearly see their hands—clenched, quiet, restless, seemingly unresponsive, or shaking.

They opened slowly over time to generously share the many lessons I have learned about caretaking and caretakers.

I wish to thank all the caretakers whose hands have shaken mine.

I want to express my deepest gratitude to my mother, for her unshakable, loving support and her voracious capacity for celebrating the life she shared with me and all those around her.

Thanks also to Zora de Bodisco, my co-author, for her patience, humor, creative writing, and editing.

Zora de Bodisco took care of her father (who had dementia during the last two years of his life) with the support of her two sisters and her wonderful husband Bill Gorman. She was instrumental in sharing her wisdom, humor, and talent in co-creating this book.

In her thirty year career with the State of Florida she received recognitions, including "Social Worker of the Year" under Florida Governor Bob Graham, and numerous innovation and achievement awards from both Health and Rehabilitative Services and the Department of Corrections.

Her early retirement was heavily weighted by the need to care for her father, who was in the early stages of dementia. She also held her aunt's hand and stuffed it with flowers and chocolates whenever she could. The roller-coaster ride that followed made the prior thirty years look tame, but she wouldn't have missed it for the world.

She is a graduate of the University of South Florida and has completed graduate work in gerontology and rehabilitation counseling.

I also wish to thank the following people: Marilyn Yergler, RN, MSN for her goodwill and editing; my husband, David Rynerson, and daughter Mia Pertik, who held my hand and my mother's hand; Bob Preble, who was one of Mom's biggest fans; and my uncle, Wadim de Bodisco, for the dignity he maintained until the end of his life despite the dementia.

Finally, I want to acknowledge the spiritual growth, influence, and inspiration of the Dalai Lama. When I while visited his temple in Dharamshala, India, I saw humility and compassion in the monks who practice compassion with all those that suffer.

I have been inspired by the work of Mother Teresa, Gandhi, and Dr. Martin Luther King, Jr., who was scheduled to march on my corner in Cicero, Illinois during the civil rights movement. At an early age, I was impacted by his life of peace, care, and compassion.

I thank all those who pursue mindfulness and kindness as a path to inner peace and life purpose.

PREFACE

The title of this book refers to reaching out, holding, and comforting with the goal of conscious compassion as a guide. Shaking hands is a form of acknowledgment.

In March 2007, my comfortable world shattered totally and permanently. All it took was a phone call from the emergency room staff at Bayfront Medical Center in St. Petersburg, Florida. My mother had been in a near-fatal car crash. I needed to come to her quickly.

As I flew from Seattle to Florida, an image played over and over again in my mind. My mother collected fragile, porcelain statues of birds. I remembered one falling through her fingers once and exploding on the floor. That is how I felt. Long after we thought all the pieces of the porcelain bird had finally been collected, another one would turn up.

Before the call, I was a Type A person, an optimistic Seattle mountain monger,

a successful therapist, a consulting regis-
tered nurse with a doctoral degree, a wife,
and a mother. After the call, my life was
shattered, and the shards were scattered
across the country.

My mother survived emergency surgery,
but it left her unable to move her hands or
legs. It was unknown if she were to remain
a quadriplegic or if this was a temporary
response to breaking her neck. She was
transferred to a rehabilitation facility and
faced a grueling recovery that would be
daunting to anyone, much less a woman
of eighty-six years.

The unraveling began. My mother and I
held hands.

Mom worked at mending physically. I
held her hand as she tried to relearn how
to walk, as we transferred her from bed to
wheelchair, while trying to stand and bathe.
Her hand held my heart, and in that way, I
could stay close to her and draw comfort
in what we shared.

When I let go, it meant that I was going back to my life in Seattle. I had to fly back and forth across the continent every other week, and like so many caretakers, I was struggling and juggling.

A few months later, Mom's physical recovery had been optimized. She declared that she wanted to leave the nursing facility and go home. Everyone thought that her days of independent living were over—everyone except for Mom, who insisted on going home. How could I manage to take care of her and keep my career in Seattle?

The unraveling process was given a name when Mom was diagnosed with Alzheimer's. It was clear when she left the rehabilitation center that she would not be able to care for herself, although she refused to acknowledge it.

I remembered a promise I'd made to my dying father in 2002 that I would always take care of my mother for him. I made the decision to gather up the pieces of my life that I could take with me and move to Florida to care for her. I had made a promise that I was committed to keeping.

Like so many with loved ones on this path, I was not surprised at the diagnosis. In some ways, it was a relief to finally come face to face with the word Mom and I had avoided. It would be a long time before I accepted the reality of Alzheimer's and longer still before I reached out with love and compassion to the shake its hand.

Before this accident Mom had continued to be willfully independent, dismissing my fears and admonishments. She ignored the minor fender benders and her increasing forgetfulness. Emotional outbursts increased, whereas always in the past she had always been even-keeled.

I had been telling her for years that her memory was fogging and she was absolutely not to drive; she could not see well due to advanced macular degeneration. Yet she aced the driving tests and her memory exam. She took the same pride in circumventing these challenges as she'd once done long ago as a survivor of World War II, leaving her home of Lithuania, fleeing the Nazis and the Communists, and surviving the work camps. In spite of all this, she earned a medical degree, became a prominent physician in Chicago, and ended her career as the medical director for tuberculosis clinics for the city of Chicago. Not bad for a woman who was penniless, stripped of her educational credentials, and unable to speak English when she arrived in the United States.

She remained a force to be reckoned with despite her illness, and she was determined to fight to keep her dignity and autonomy. After a lifetime of overcoming tribulation, the insurmountable Elena Pertik was not going to give up without the fight of her life.

Bit by bit, she lost the fight. Her mind slipped away, though she never openly admitted that anything was wrong. To admit a problem was to admit loss of control and acknowledge her fears.

Florida was hot and flat, compared to the vibrant Olympic mountains and amethyst Puget Sound of Seattle. The abrupt closure of a thriving practice and the hasty goodbyes to lifelong friends left me disoriented and lonely, but I told myself that I was only as good as my word.

Despite my attempts at planning, nothing could have prepared me for the responsibility of my mother's well-being. Because she was entirely incapacitated and obviously in mental and emotional distress, our roles were reversed. I felt like I was struggling to parent a willful, eighty-six-year-old toddler. The woman I had always relied on as a beacon of strength now trusted me with her life and exasperated me at every turn.

I told myself that I was in for better or worse as I danced around her moods.

It got much worse. I juggled trying to accept to what I'd been forced to leave behind—my home, support system, college-age daughter, husband, career—and adjust to my now long-distance family, establishing a new career, and making new friends. I did all this while taking care of Mom.

The situation felt impossible, but I had made a promise that I would be my mother's caretaker, and I was determined to keep that promise. I told myself I would just learn to juggle better, faster, and more efficiently, and I tried to do just that.

In the meantime, I lived apart from my husband, who was working in another state. I missed my only daughter's college graduation. The house I'd always seen as my refuge was put up for sale and then burglarized. My body crumbled from the stress, and I developed aches, pains, and symptoms I had never had before. My morning coffee was accompanied by migraine headaches and cervical neck pain.

My future looked dark. I wondered who would live longer—my Mom or me? As I became more angry, resentful, depressed, and guilty, she seemed less resentful and happier to get my attention.

I loved my mother with all my heart, but what I was doing was breaking me down, breaking down my family, and breaking down everything I'd worked so hard for.

What was I doing? Why I was doing this?

From somewhere within me, a voice calmly said, "It is in the giving that you receive." I did not know it at the time but have since learned that this was a verse from the Bible.

Give, and it will be given to you.
A good measure, pressed down, shaken
together and running over, will be poured
into your lap. For with the measure
you use, it will be measured to you.
Luke 6:38

Slowly my situation changed —not miraculously, in a bright flash of light. Don't we all wish that were how it worked?

Change came slowly but in small measured steps. I began a journal in which I recorded the time with my mom, my fears, and my hopes. Sometimes one day of madness and frustration ran hopelessly into the next, but I began to recognize the dark moments and how I overcame them. More importantly, I recognized the good moments and celebrated them.

I searched for support, joined support groups, and learned that I was not alone. I came to realize that I had never been alone—I just did not know how to reach out.

I set my alarm for 4:00 a.m. so that I could read and pray before Mom woke up. I knew my day would be full once Mom needed me, so I took a tiny piece of the morning for myself. I tried to read spiritual material while on the StairMaster to sneak in as much self-care as I could.

I joined a mediation and prayer group, where some members were in similar predicaments, and I was amazed at how many people were involved in or affected by Alzheimer's. This allowed me to find support when I needed it and to take time to reflect.

I was actively searching for comfort and answers. If they were there, I wanted to find them, and in making that my intention, I began to regain my strength and balance.

My search led me to the belief that life naturally brings suffering and that out of desperation, our life journey evolves and personal transformation occurs. In one of my support groups, I was told that this is "the gift of despair." I was told, "Have faith, and the miracle of seeing the light in the journey will appear."

I want to share what worked for me with you. The seven steps in this book evolved from my pain, mistakes, accomplishments, and what I learned from other caretakers. Through the lessons learned by the caring for my mother, I began to find ease rather than dis-ease.

I gathered information by listening to other caregivers, bankers, police officers, emergency room doctors, assisted living administrators, mental health professionals, family members, and people with Alzheimer's.

As my beliefs shifted, so did the quality of my life. I began to experience moments of deep serenity and gratitude. The more I practiced my spiritual fitness, the less spiritual "indigestion" I felt. I no longer felt like a victim. I stopped blaming my mother. I learned that my happiness is solely dependent on my willingness to experience the healing energy of compassion.

People I have met with Alzheimer's have been my teachers, and hence the handshakes continue. I wrote this book because I believe that in teaching and holding close, I learned what I needed to learn. Being a humble, compassionate person was a choice that I could repel or embrace.

I chose to embrace compassion. It brought me closer to my own healing and ultimately my own well-being.

Before I finished this book, Mom died peacefully in her own home, in her own bed. I am grateful for this, because it was what she deeply wanted. I kept my promise to her, to my father, and to myself.

The wisdom I heard in a moment of despair helped me find my learning path and find that it is indeed in giving that I receive.

With gratitude, I now gladly give what I have learned on this path to you.

INTRODUCTION

Alzheimer's reaches out and directly shakes our hands. We don't recognize its grasp, because we expect it to come with gray hair and a Medicare card.

Our neck stiffens a bit when we hear Mom laughingly explain that they were late for the annual family picnic because Dad forgot how to get to the park.

Alzheimer's grasp is in the small hand of a first grader who is frightened of his dear Mami—she once adored him and now slaps him away. He wants to know what he has done wrong and why she does not love him anymore.

It challenges us in the clenched fist of a teenager who cannot explain why hanging out in the streets is preferable to doing home-work in a house that reeks of his uncle's urine.

It comes in the frustration of the over-stretched small business owner being handed yet another Family Medical Leave

Act form and wishing that she had never hired the person who had seemed to be a promising employee.

Alzheimer's hands the overwhelmed caretaker a fine martini, and then another, and another, and perhaps pain pills to "help ease the pain."

It picks the pockets of law enforcement agencies stretching precious dollars in Silver Alerts and trying to locate patients who have wandered away from home or from an assisted living facility and from dispatchers and emergency personnel who answer endless 911 calls from a confused person who remembers only that number to call for help.

Alzheimer's emerges in the vomit outside a home where an elderly woman is found tied to a bed in a back bedroom, maggots crawling over her bedsores.

Who would do such a thing? The demented monster who restrained his mother in such an inhumane fashion should be prosecuted and thrown in prison. The "monster" is a mentally challenged son who is trying to keep Mama safe because she keeps wandering away and might get hurt. His hands tied love knots. Are there enough hands in social service programs, judicial systems, and support agencies to reach out to him?

Will the postman question the increasing number of "prize winning notifications" and charitable requests filling the mailbox of the person with Alzheimer's on his route, or will he simply hand them over? What about the "friends" that appear only when the Social Security checks arrive?

Who is able to grasp the extent of the damage done by those who victimize their own trusting parents and loved ones through shady deals and money transfers, while promising that they will be cared for and allowed to die in dignity?

Are there enough vigilant and proactive investment firms, banks, and financial institutions to stop this victimization?

We shake the hand of Alzheimer's whether we like it or not.

As you read this, you may have thought of a family member, neighbor, co-worker, student, or employee that struggles with this disease.

Do you feel differently now?

If you still do not think Alzheimer's directly affects you, think of the billions of tax dollars spent on the disease. Billions on top of that are spent in social services and law enforcement. The costs of businesses, education, and collateral institutions multiply and spread through added costs in products and services.

The recent health care-related cases amount to approximately $172 billion and the number is rising. The statistics are increasing daily.

We are in the middle of an epidemic. While efforts focus on research, diagnosis, medication, technology, facilities, and prevention, few researchers are studying how "compassionate caregiving" affects those with Alzheimer's.

Alzheimer's affects about five million people in the United States. One in six people over sixty-five will be diagnosed with Alzheimer's and one in two persons over eighty-five. Alzheimer's is being diagnosed earlier and in younger people (currently, two hundred thousand people under the age of sixty have Alzheimer's).

Every seventy seconds, someone is diagnosed with Alzheimer's, and in forty years, the rate will drop to every thirty-three seconds. The number of patients will more than double. In the United States, someone turns sixty years old every six seconds. In forty years, there will be nineteen million Americans age eighty-five and older. All of these people will need a hired caretaker or a family member to provide services for them.

Seventy percent of those with Alzheimer's live at home, and they yearn for the person who helps them to be kind and patient. They hope that the health-care provider, banker, and pharmacist will understand them, and they need the tender compassion that dwells within all of us.

The Purpose of This Book

This book will help any caretaker to be mindful of the power of compassion when dealing with a person with Alzheimer's. This book is purposely simple. Caretakers are pressed for time, and the steps for compassion are simple. All it takes is a sincere desire to embody the noblest gesture.

It is only through practice and application that our busy lives are transformed into compassionate ones.

This book is intended for the following individuals:

1. Persons seeking a guide on compassionate caregiving for an Alzheimer's patient and how to apply the principles on their own or in a group setting.
2. Persons who work in assisted living facilities, financial institutions, health-care settings, medical

offices, hospitals, rehabilitation centers, law enforcement, and academic settings as well as attorneys and mental health professionals.
3.   Persons whose own lives have been touched by compassion and who wish to pass on the gift.

Suggestions for Using This Book

In the chapters that follow, I outline seven steps. Consider completing one step each week: this provides a mindset to absorb what you are embracing.

1.   Read the step.
2.   Go to the self-awareness/assessment tool.
3.   Practice the exercise and activity for applying what you have read.
4.   Use self-observation and reflection.
5.   Seal the step with the affirmations.
6.   Repeat the breathing and affirmations often during the day.

Useful Terms

Breathing: Awareness of the breath is emphasized in this book. Focus on the breath is the landing pad for an easily distracted mind. It highlights awareness of air as it goes into the body through the nostrils and /or mouth. Breathing connects us to now, the present moment—not the past or the future. Focusing on now relaxes the mind and allows the body to relax. The heart slows, the muscles relax, and we feel an overall sense of well-being.

Affirmations: Focused thoughts and language that are directed toward one's well-being.

Self-awareness tool: A self-assessment that guides the caretaker toward greater awareness.

Benefit: The positive results from mastering and putting the step into practice.

"Accept the things to which fate binds you, and love the people with whom fate brings you together, but do so with all your heart." ——Marcus Aurelius

WHAT IS ALZHEIMER'S DISEASE?

Alzheimer's is one form of dementia. There are many others, but it is the most common type of irreversible dementia. The cause of Alzheimer's is still unknown, but age, health habits, and genetics play a significant role.

Alzheimer's is a disease of the brain. The brain is the master control center of the body; it is made up of billions of cells called neurons and has a huge network of blood vessels. The brain receives 20 percent of the body's blood supply, which carries oxygen, glucose (sugar), and other nutrients and hormones needed for normal functioning.

Alzheimer's destroys the brain by killing brain cells. It begins as the abnormal plaques and tangles start to develop, which might occur years before the disease is diagnosed. It is known that the amyloid precursor protein (APP) is the starting point for the sticky plaques, and certain enzymes can cause it to fragment and clump.

The brains of individuals with Alzheimer's have abundant sticky tangles and plaques (the deposits of protein fragments). They result in a predictable pattern of changes, usually starting with memory loss, personality changes and behavioral changes such as impulsiveness, agitation, anxiety, combativeness, withdrawal. Forgetting daily tasks becomes increasingly noticeable.

Alzheimer's is slowly progressive. It is irreversible, and there is no cure. Those with Alzheimer's live an average of eight years after their symptoms become noticeable to other people, but they can survive up to twenty years or longer, depending on how early the onset was and other health conditions.

For practical purposes, I will divide the pattern of Alzheimer's disease into three stages.

Early Stage

Most people in early stage Alzheimer's may be able to live at home unless safety issues such as getting lost are noted. There is a noticeable loss of spontaneity due to fear of getting lost; changing the predictable familiarity of the person's home environment causes anxiety. Speech is somewhat impaired, as the person may use some words inappropriately or forget the meaning of some words. A slight effort to communicate and understand what a conversation is about may be apparent. Stories may be repeated.

The first noticeable challenges are typically about finances, such as balancing a checkbook. Poor judgment may lead to financial concerns. A problem having to do with banking often alerts family members that something is not right.

Patients may increasingly lose or misplace objects like keys or a wallet and have difficulty organizing their daily activities. They may forget something that they just read and show impulsive behaviors that are atypical for them. Their short-term memory is compromised, and their confusion increases.

Changes in routines—such as house guests, travel, or leaving familiar surroundings—may cause agitation.

Beyond these symptoms, the person with early stage Alzheimer's may seem completely healthy. However, more and more effort is spent denying that anything is wrong. Because they fear a diagnosis of Alzheimer's, both the patient and the family members can live in a state of denial, which can prevent them from seeking medical and psychological assessment and treatment.

Middle Stage

At this stage, the patient's short-term memory becomes increasingly worse. Where in the early stage of Alzheimer's car keys may frequently be lost, now patients may forget what the car keys are used for. Their speech may become impaired, and they may use words inappropriately. Their frustration increases as they are unable to understand what is being said to them (such as instructions for a specific task).

Repetition of stories or actions becomes more noticeable.

Personality differences become markedly noticeable, particularly as the use of vulgar language may emerge. The patient may become more anxious, restless, repetitive, withdrawn, and forgetful; illogical thinking is more evident.

Changes in behavior may manifest themselves in the late afternoon or evening. This has led to the term "Sundowner's Syndrome.

Some patients may experience hallucinations and feel suspicious of others. They may see people from the past and think that they themselves are in the past.

They have more problems with performing complex tasks, such as managing their finances, and they may forget recent events. A person with Alzheimer's may go to her granddaughter's sixteenth birthday party and immediately afterward not remember having attended.

Safety is a major issue during this stage, as six out of ten people with Alzheimer's will wander off and become lost. This typically alarms the family member, fire fighter, law enforcement officer, banker, grocery store, and neighbors. At this point, the need for a caretaker must be addressed, and getting help is paramount.

Late Stage

The end stage of the disease is focused on comfort care. Both short-term and long-term memory are significantly altered. The patients cannot recognize family and loved ones, which can be excruciatingly painful for the family members who have cared for them. They are unable to eat, or sometimes even move. Patients in end stage Alzheimer's may see the car and the car keys and not know what either of them is used for. They are unable to recall their address, what day it is, or what clothing to wear for the season or occasion.

In the final stages of the disease, they may lose the ability to respond to normal stimulation, to smile, or to hold their head up without support. Their reflexes become abnormal, and their muscles go rigid. Swallowing is impaired, choking is a hazard, and they may lose weight due to the inability to eat. They may have skin infections from loss of bowel or bladder control. A person in end-stage Alzheimer's often loses the ability to speak and may only groan. This is the end of life with Alzheimer's disease.

"Wherever you go, go with all your heart."——Confucius

WHAT IS COMPASSION?

Compassion is love. Compassion is tenderness and a sincere desire to have a positive response toward the person with Alzheimer's. It is a deep awareness of the suffering of another, coupled with the wish to relieve that suffering. It comes from empathy and consideration of the well-being of others. It stems from the heart and guides us to do the work of being caretakers. It spurs the desire in the caretaker to develop skills to alleviate the suffering and provide comfort.

While compassion is a look inward, the actions are expressed outwardly through service. It is gentle and kind, and it is where true transformation and our own healing take place. The mindfulness of compassion allows us to live with an attitude of gratitude and share that joy with others. Compassion is something we all desire, regardless of age, race, or socioeconomic level. It is seeing the commonality between us and bypassing differences.

Throughout history, we have turned to compassionate teachers in times of turmoil. As examples of true compassion, I think of Jesus, Buddha, Mother Teresa, Martin Luther King, Jr., Gandhi, and the Dalai Lama.

Compassion is immediately felt and understood. It is what the patients with Alzheimer's respond to and feel, and it is what they are starving for.

When I see a caretaker of someone who has Alzheimer's, I empathize with the caregiver's journey and what that entails. When I see a person with Alzheimer's, I see my own mother again. As people that I have told about this book have shared their stories with me, I understand how vulnerable they feel.

Compassion requires conviction and a commitment to make a choice to be positive to self and others. Adopting a sense of caring brings inner strength and joy.

Compassion has no boundaries when it comes to caring. It does not discriminate or judge. Its emblem is an open mind and heart.

"*I cannot be everything to everyone.*
I just hope that I am something
to someone." ——*Anonymous*

"*You can give without loving, but you can't*
love without giving." —— *Anonymous*

STEP ONE: INTENTIONAL COMPASSION

Reflect on your intentions for being a caretaker.

Intention may be defined like this: "To have a purpose and a focused mind."

Intention is understanding what your purpose is and why you are doing what you are doing. Intention keeps you on track. It is the foundation of our sense of who we are, and examining our motives allows us to be aware of ourselves.

It is vital to know specifically why you choose to care for a person with Alzheimer's. When you are aware of yourself, you become aware of how your choices directly impact the course of your experience as a caretaker and what the person experiences when with you. Knowing your intentions is the first step.

This book is about being conscious of your genuine motivations, and this awareness will allow you to feel the positive effects of compassion each time you think about it. Merely thinking good thoughts changes your biochemistry. It releases oxytocin, sometimes called the "love hormone," which is the hormone released when mothers bond with their newborn. It enables brain cells to mirror other's brain cells so that your behavior directly affects another person's behavior. In this way, people respond to compassion and empathy.

Being aware of your intention is also necessary to monitor your own state of mind and thoughts. How you direct your mind stems directly from your intention and sense of purpose.

The average human has approximately 240 thoughts per minute, so be clear about what those thoughts are about when you are a caretaker. These thoughts unearth your intentions and carry you through the good times and the bad times.

When I speak to caretakers of people with Alzheimer's, I hear mostly that they love their role and work. They love the person they are caring for. I also hear some care-takers say that they do not have a choice: their family has no one else, they feel guilty, it's the only job they could find, they need the money, and so on.

If you base your caretaking experience on resentment, guilt, anger, frustration, or disgust, you have thousands of negative thoughts per day. That flood of negativity impacts both you and the person with Alzheimer's, and it will eventually burn you out. If you try to override the negativity, it will pop up somewhere else, out of nowhere.

Negativity can make you ill in all realms of life, mentally, physically and spiritually. It erodes your life, and the person with Alzheimer's can feel it. It makes the patient unhappy and more agitated.

Knowing what your intentions are and reminding yourself of them during difficult times will maintain focus about the positives of your experience as a caretaker.

The first step is about looking within yourself and determining to be conscious of your intention as a gentle caretaker. You are in control of what you think, and your intentions show you the way in difficult situations. Love and compassion melt the hardest situations. Compassion breaks down the walls of isolation and brings peace of mind.

Once you can define your intention, you can remind yourself of your purpose and align your experiences with your thoughts. Unconscious choices occur before you are aware of them, so you can be a negative, reactive zombie or a positive, free-willed, compassionate caretaker.

STEP ONE: SELF-AWARENESS TOOL

❖ Do you get impatient when you hear repeated questions and remarks from the person with Alzheimer's?

❖ Do you find yourself angry when the person with Alzheimer's says? " No" to any of your suggestions?

❖ Do you resent cleaning up after the person with Alzheimer's?

❖ Do you resent how much time the person with Alzheimer's is taking from your life?

If you answered yes to any of these questions, evaluate whether being a caretaker is the best decision for you.

Taking care of someone with Alzheimer's is a challenge, and finding another caretaker or facility that meets his or her needs and personality can be a true act of compassion.

If caretaking isn't working for you, talk to someone about your role and what you can do to feel better about being a caretaker. A multitude of resources are available, including those at the back of this book.

Many people feel guilt about having their family member moved to an assisted living facility, but being a caretaker is an extremely difficult job and not suited for everyone regardless of their desires. Asking for help is a sign of strength. For example, some people are good at accounting (I am not one of those gifted people). At tax time, I need to ask for help with my accounting. Our lives are not "one size fits all." We have our authentic contributions, and being a caretaker may not be for you or it may be for you. An honest inventory of your motives helps clarify your direction.

It is an act of compassion to see that the person with Alzheimer's lives in a safe, loving environment, where his or her needs can be met. If your intention is to give your family member the best that you can, make a choice to let go of guilt.

STEP ONE: EXERCISE

We are the sum total of our choices, and behind every choice is an intention, a belief system. It is this "seed thought" that determines our actions.

List five of your intentions for being a caretaker.

1.
2.
3.
4.
5.

When a person is not able to take care of an Alzheimer's patient, it is important to know that letting the patient be taken care by another person or an assisted living home is an act of compassion.

KARLA'S STORY-

Karla took care of her much older sister, Pam, who had Alzheimer's. Karla told me that anger and frustration were seeping into all areas of her life. She did not have enough patience to slow down to interact with Pam. She felt resentful that she could not do anything right for Pam, and that Pam had ruined her family life.

Karla was the office manager for a small business, and her self-esteem was based on being a competent high achiever and a solution person. She said, "I was always the one that would took care of every problem—that is why I managed my office like a tight-running ship. Now I cannot stand my sister. Now I sit in my car in the garage and scream."

Karla's college-age daughter sat down with her and told her that Auntie Pam might get more interaction in an assisted living facility. She asked, "Mom why are you doing this? It's killing you and destroying our family." After hearing this from her own daughter, Karla began to weep. "I am a failure. I cannot even take care of my own sister!"

She realized that her intentions were based on guilt. She was motivated to take care of her sister only because she felt she had no other options. Given her can-do personality, she felt that caring for Pam was something she had to do or else she was "a failure." After some brutal soul-searching, she realized that Pam would be much better off living where other people could give her the time and attention that she needed.

After spending time looking at various facilities with Pam, they found a facility near Karla's house that was a good fit for everyone. They could play Bingo together, and Pam could come to Karla's house and help in the garden. Pam gained weight, was interacting more, and was able to say that she did not feel like a burden to Karla. Pam, Karla, and her entire family were happier. Finding a facility that met Pam's needs was an act of compassion.

Karla let go of her perception of her self-worth being dependent on being Pam's caretaker. She made a conscious choice for Pam's well-being with honor and respect, and she let go of ego and guilt.

If guilt and resentment are your motivations for being a caretaker and you feel you are taken for granted and taken advantage of, it will cause a great deal of suffering for the caretaker and the person with Alzheimer's. Allowing someone else with a disposition suited for caretaking is a loving, kind, compassionate gesture.

Resentment is a poison that creates a negative atmosphere and serves no purpose other than making people miserable and ill. Some people look at their work begrudgingly, while some people see giving as an opportunity to be of service to their loved ones or residents. Love and compassion are contagious. If we are focused on being loving people in a loving world, and that being a caretaker is a privilege, our experience will be one of love, kindness, and tolerance.

STEP ONE: BREATHING EXERCISE

You will see a repitition and some variation of this breathing exercise throughout the steps. Use this often, and it will become an automatic response. This mindfulness of your breathing will bring oxygen to your brain, slow your heart rate and give you a frame of mind that is compassionate for your mind and heart.

BEFORE you begin any breathing exercise first pay attention to how you are breathing and what you are feeling at the moment.

Find a quiet place where you can be alone for at least a few moments. It can be outside by a pond or in a bathroom stall at your office. You just don't want to be disturbed.

Close your eyes and begin to breathe in deeply and slowly. Breathe through your nose or mouth, which ever feels most natural to you.

As you inhale connect with your feeling by clearly naming it. Many times our feelings seem to swirl around us in confusion, especially in emotionally charged situations.

When you name the feeling you are stopping that emotional "overload" of free floating anxiety and thoughts.

Now that you have named the feeling (love, hurt, compassion, frustration, joy) allow it to expand as the air fills your lungs.

Let the feeling grow larger and larger.

Let it fill you entirely and as it does allow yourself to focus deeply on the feeling.

Imagine it flowing throughout your body along with the oxygen you are inhaling and let it travel until it has reached the tips of your fingers, the top of your head, the soles of your feet, and behind your closed eyes.

Now slowly release your breath through your nose or your mouth, whichever is more comfortable.

As you exhale, release the feeling along with your breath.

Feel it slipping out.

Empty your body of it - let it go.

As you do, can you sense the parts of your body that suddenly feel lighter? Less tense? Somehow emptied?

This exercise can work in very powerful ways whether dealing with positive of negative emotions, or even the feeling of being overwhelmed, because all emotions can be stressful until acknowledged and directed.

Since this **first step breathing exercise** focuses on our **intentions** in being a caretaker go back to your intentions list and pick an emotion you listed. For example, you may have written "I love my mom so much" or "I resent being a caretaker because no one else would."

Pick one word you associate as an emotion for that statement. Is it love? Loss? Anger? Joy? Compassion?

Now that you have named the emotion, begin the breathing exercise again.

STEP ONE: AFFIRMATIONS

Start with your full inhalation breath and exhale, stating the affirmation out loud, sealed with a smile.

"I am a loving person in a loving world."
"I am a compassionate person with all my intentions."
"My intentions stem from compassion."
"Compassion gives me serenity."

STEP ONE: BENEFITS

Being aware of your intentions for being a caretaker encourages you to be proactive rather than reactive. Reminding yourself of your intentions allows you to focus on your compassionate self. Using breathing exercises and affirmations allow you to reinforce the positive aspects of caregiving as well as relieve the inevitable stress of the role. This brings serenity. You are able to detach and be kind and loving.

For the next week spend time absorbing what you have taken from step one and build on the skills you have started to develop. Review your intentions list. You will likely be surprised to see that you have changed or added to it as the week progresses. That's fine, it is meant to be part of growth and self-awareness. You may already find yourself automatically falling into controlled breathing and the use of positive affirmation.

"You can't change the past, but you can ruin a perfectly good present by trying to control the future." —Maria *"DR MO"* Pertik

STEP TWO: LET GO OF THE NEED TO CONTROL

I often hear caretakers say, "I feel powerless."

LAURA'S STORY-

Laura told me "As mom's disease progressed, I felt utterly powerless. I became overly controlling to the point of becoming blind to the light of compassion. The more she became combative and agitated, refusing to bathe, eat, or do things I thought she would enjoy, the more I was driven to try to rescue her. The more chaotic things got, the more my response was to become obsessive, trying to convince her and direct her to the task at hand.

Mom said to me once, 'There has to be more in my life other than being pushed and pulled around, doing what you want me to be doing.' This showed up in everything I did. I built an addition to my house, got new furniture, and bought clothes for Mom, things that she could put on and take off easily. This backfired in a big way.

Mom refused to wear anything I got her, did not go anywhere I suggested, and it was as though she went on a hunger strike.

I created a schedule, scoured the community for activities Mom would love such as the beach, stamp collecting, and the senior center. The more I did, the more resistance I got."

Laura was exhausted.

When I visit with other caretakers, I see them "guiding, pushing, pulling, and rushing." This approach is certain to backfire on you. As I was teaching a class on Alzheimer's in a facility, I heard one of the caretakers say, "Hell is truth seen too late." The more you try to control people with Alzheimer's, the more they will resist.

More controlling = more resistance = loss of compassion = loss of serenity

Fear and Anxiety

I felt great fear and anxiety over the notion that I was out of control while watching my mother deteriorate before my eyes and I overcompensated by being controlling. I needed to feel that I could control all the tasks of daily living and had this notion that unless everything was done for her, she would never be happy. It became an obsession.

In my mind, I was a good caretaker when I prepared meals, shopped, managed finances, kept track of the mounting medical bills, managed legal affairs, helped Mom use her walker or wheelchair which she forgot she needed for bathing, dressing, and feeding, helped her use the toilet, cleaned up accidents of incontinence, took her to medical visits, and scheduled social activities and outings. The lists never ended.

There is no way that I could do all these things alone. When Mom had outbursts (and predictably she did any time I tried to rush her), my controlling attitude slowed everything down. The more I rushed and tried to control, the more resistance Mom gave me.

Another mistake I made was changing Mom's home and furniture when she was in the hospital. I repainted the walls and removed the clutter. This was a terrible thing to do for someone with Alzheimer's, and it was another example of the need to control. Even though I thought the new paint and furniture would be cheerful changes that she would welcome, they were disrespectful of what Mom really enjoyed.

I lost sight of my intention and became a robotic taskmaster. My sense of self-worth was directly correlated to the tasks I had gotten done.

The truth is that caregivers are powerless over the mental and functional losses that come with Alzheimer's. We can control only our responses and ourselves. Acceptance and focusing on compassion are the keys to serenity.

TIM'S STORY-

Tim inspired me to create the exercise for Step Two. Tim was an attorney and was seen as a "helper." He worked for the county as a public defender and as a troubleshooter. In his mind, he was good at cleaning up messes. He was knowledgeable and took pride in being able to fix complex cases that came to him.

His youth and life with his family was a troubled one. However, when it came time to make a decision about who would take care of his father (who had been abusive to him and his siblings when they were children), Tim thought he was obviously the person best able to do so. Tim tried to control his father when he wandered away from the house and became distraught when his father did not do what he asked. His father began to not recognize him, adding to Tim's feelings of being out of control.

Tim admitted that he was an "addicted fixer upper of other people's problems." Tim became more controlling and said it felt like he was going insane because he could not "fix" his father. The more he tried to "manage" his father, the more resistant his father became. Tim became enmeshed with his father's behavior, depressed, and unable to emotionally detach. When he went to his pastor for help, it was pointed out this was a very unhealthy way of thinking, feeling, and acting.

Tim realized that he was not in control of his father's behavior or Alzheimer's. He let go of the need to have the answers, to prevent erratic behavior, or to try to act "together" when he was falling apart. He let go of his enmeshment with the role of being in control, being the person who could do miracles for his father. Tim was able to admit that his motivation for control was a yearning for approval and recognition from his father, brother, sister, and estranged extended family. Everyone in his family walked away from their father when the money ran out except for Tim.

When Tim realized that he could not control the disease, and that he could control only his own choices and how he thought about himself, his father, and Alzheimer's, the anxiety lifted from his shoulders. He said, "I began calling my brother and sister and delegating things that they could do to help Dad. I did not take any excuse for not pitching in as a team effort, and I let go of my pride that only I can control and fix my dad."

STEP TWO: SELF-AWARENESS TOOL

❖ Do you feel tension when you are not in total control?
❖ Do you have a need for certainty?
❖ Do you feel a need to predict everything that will occur during the day?
❖ Do you feel like you have to complete everything on your to do list before you can relax?

If you answered yes to more than one of these questions, it is time to try Step Two.

STEP TWO: SELF AWARENESS EXERCISE

List all the things you can control in your life.

List all the things you can control with Alzheimer's as the disease progresses.

Describe the times when you think a person with Alzheimer's is happy or peaceful.

Do these situations relate to your need to maintain control?

STEP TWO: BREATHING EXERCISE

NOTE: You will see a variation of this breathing exercise throughout the steps after a reminder of how to do the exercise. As you become familiar with controlled breathing by doing it often, it will become an automatic response and you will not need to read these preliminary directions and can just go forward to the exercise specific to this step.

This mindfulness of your breathing will bring oxygen to your brain, slow your heart rate and give you a frame of mind that is compassionate for your mind and heart.

BEFORE you begin any breathing exercise first pay attention to how you are breathing and what you are feeling at the moment.

Find a quiet place where you can be alone for at least a few moments. It can be outside by a pond or in a bathroom stall at your office. You just don't want to be disturbed.

Close your eyes and begin to breathe in deeply and slowly. Breathe through your nose or mouth, which ever feels most natural to you.

As you inhale connect with your feeling by clearly naming it. Many times our feelings seem to swirl around us in confusion, especially in emotionally charged situations.

When you name the feeling you are stopping that emotional "overload".

Now that you have named the feeling (love, hurt, compassion, frustration, joy), allow it to expand as the air fills your lungs.

Let the feeling grow larger and larger.

Let it fill you entirely and as it does allow yourself to focus deeply on the feeling.

Imagine it flowing throughout your body along with the oxygen you are inhaling and let it travel until it has reached the tips of your fingers, the top of your head, the soles of your feet, and behind your closed eyes.

Now slowly release your breath through your nose or your mouth, whichever is more comfortable.

As you exhale, release the feeling along with your breath.

Feel it slipping out.

Empty your body of it - let it go.

As you do, can you sense the parts of your body that suddenly feel lighter? Less tense? Somehow emptied?

This exercise can work in very powerful ways, whether dealing with positive of negative emotions or even the feeling of being overwhelmed, because all emotions can be stressful until acknowledged and directed.

The **second step breathing exercise** focuses on our need to **give up control.** Spend a moment thinking of being out of control and how it feels for you. What is one word you would use to describe what you are feeling? Do you feel frightened? Angry? Anxious? Humiliated?

Now that you have named the emotion, begin the breathing exercise.

A BONUS exercise for step two is one called REHEARSAL.
A technique I use whenever I want to be prepared for any behavior change is called "Rehearsal." It is mentally imagining what

you want to actually do. This technique is also sometimes called creative visualization.

Imagine a situation where you have tried to control the person with Alzheimer's and the person resisted your efforts. Perhaps it is getting her to bathe, eat, or change clothes.

Try to imagine it as clearly as you can with all your senses. Can you see the situation? Smell it? Hear it?

Notice how you feel and react when she is not cooperating with you.

Again, use your senses. Are your muscles tightening? Where? Does your jaw tighten? Do you feel warm? What smells do you smell? What feelings are you feeling? Exhausted? Are you crying? Angry?

Now imagine yourself breathing in, and as you breathe out, say, "I let go of the need to control."

Imagine sitting down and being compassionate, acting with love and kindness. Notice yourself relaxing as you do this. Notice her relaxing when you do this.

Imagine that you are acknowledging what she is telling you and listening with your heart.

What do you hear her say to you? What do you sense about her needs without words? How did you sense this?

STEP TWO: AFFIRMATIONS

Breathe in and out again, and say to yourself: "I choose to let go of the need to control." "I choose compassion over my need to control."

STEP TWO: BENEFITS

Letting go gives us freedom from the need to feel in control. The reality is that you cannot control the progression of Alzheimer's, only your reaction to it. Letting go of control opens up your experience of compassion, which makes you feel better about yourself and what you are doing. The person you are caring for is also freed from the bondage of an environment that feels frightening and restricting.

Remember:

**More controlling = more resistance
= loss of compassion = loss of serenity**

For the next week spend time absorbing what you have taken from step two and build on the skills you are developing. The need for control is a difficult one for caretakers who often face pulls from many different directions and is so bound to our self-esteem. In this step you have acknowledged some personal needs that may bind you to controlling and started developing tools to pick apart those knots.

Maria Pertik

BE HERE NOW!

STEP THREE: VALIDATION AS COMPASSION

Validation is communication with an Alzheimer's patient that focuses on feelings rather than factual content. It is not about the words but about the emotion.

We show that we care by truly listening. We listen by stopping our agenda of tasks, waiting for the person with Alzheimer's to finish what they are saying, paying attention to verbal and non-verbal communication and maybe even taking notes.

As Alzheimer's progresses, patients lose short-term memory. They can also lose the ability to verbally express themselves and to understand the words said to them.

Imagine not knowing where you are and trying to connect with the stranger in front of you (the caretaker) who is trying to remove your clothes for a shower!

The irony is that long-term memory becomes everyday reality. While caretakers unsuccessfully try to connect to the present and the tasks at hand (such as taking a shower or going to eat breakfast), the patient may become more confused and frustrated because "today's tasks" are not reality. The caretaker's efforts are frightening.

In a healthy brain, short-term memory is intact, and we can use the thinking and the sequencing portions of the brain to tell the difference between the past and present. The person with Alzheimer's cannot.

The art of validation is going into the patient's world whatever it may be, acknowledging it verbally, and mirroring what he communicates to us.

We validate by pausing to wait for the patients to finish what they are saying—some can write or draw what they are trying to communicate. We may use a picture board for expressions (such as a sad face or a happy face). A picture of a toilet, a sofa, a plate of food, or a loved one may help him to express to the caretaker what is going on inside of him.

By attempting and acknowledging the connection with him, we show him that we are listening with the true intention of compassion.

Validation is listening, not arguing. The person with Alzheimer's is trying to tell us his truth. If he loses his ability to verbally express himself, he is acting out his experience of his truth, and it is absolutely true for him, no matter how far-fetched it may sound. What he tells us is true and "in the now" for him. This is the true meaning of "be here now." Look beyond the words and dive into the feelings being expressed.

The skill of validation means accepting, entering, and acknowledging the world of the person with Alzheimer's. If the feelings are not acknowledged, they will gather strength, and the person will act out even more forcefully to try to get his feelings across.

A caregiver named Marlow told me this story. "I met a man who refused to change his clothes. He would carry a stuffed animal—a cat—around with him. When I would try to change his soiled clothes, he would cry. I told him that the cat had had an 'accident' on his pants and soiled them and needed to be changed as soon as possible. He responded, 'Oh yes indeed!' and cooperated and took the clothes off."

Here is another example. A man named Arthur started taking off his clothes in a recreational therapy room that had blue carpeting. His wife asked him, "Arthur, what are you doing?" Arthur replied, "I am going swimming in the pool right here in front of me". His wife walked away for a minute, then came back and said to him, "The lifeguard is off duty, and the pool is being cleaned for regular maintenance." Arthur replied, "Okay then, I can swim tomorrow." He zipped up his pants and walked away.

Arthur's wife validated his experience by acknowledging that he saw the pool. After validating his experience, she shifted his attention and stopped him from undressing further.

Here is a hypothetical scenario. Imagine that you are a caregiver at Serenity Acres Assisted Living Facility. Gloria is a daycare resident who wants to talk about her husband, Bill, who died ten years ago. You have planned a day on the beach looking for shells and dinner at the Coastline Café. Suddenly Gloria becomes anxious and frantic. Bill is supposed to bring the boat around for a fishing trip. Your discussion of shells and tonight's dinner is not reality for Gloria, and she is not interested in your plan. As she looks for Bill, she becomes more anxious. You can validate her feelings by focusing on her agenda instead of yours. Your method of validation could be something like this:

"Oh, you are waiting for Bill to get the boat."

"Tell me about the boat."

"What does it look like?"

"Is Bill a good fisherman?"

You validate what Gloria said by repeating her statement. You asked her to tell you more about what she was concerned about and what she is experiencing.

A note of caution: While these statements validate the person's experience, the intention is not to "rapid fire" the questions, which could easily make the situation worse. After the first statement, wait, listen to the response, and decide where to go from there.

Telling Gloria that her husband is dead would be shocking, as he is alive and well in her reality. Telling Gloria that she is at your outing and that you are going to the Coastline Cafe when she is looking for a boat would agitate her. How might you react if you were Gloria and I tell you about the outing I've planned and that we are going to the Coastline Café even though your husband is missing? Spend time listening to Gloria and what she has to say, even though it is not based on your reality.

Validation is acknowledging what Gloria is saying, never arguing about what you think is reality, because the more you argue, the more she will argue back that she needs to find her husband Bill. Arguing with a person who has Alzheimer's serves no purpose. You will terrify them and agitate them.

The person with Alzheimer's is always right. Validation is moving into their world and freeing your imagination to join their world. Repeat what they tell you, ask questions about it, and acknowledge their perceptions and feelings about what is happening. If you choose not to do this, the patient will not stop trying to convince you about what he is experiencing. It can become a circular argument that ends in distress.

I used to attempt to convince my mother of the here and now, and I said what might be one of the cruelest remarks to someone with Alzheimer's: "Mom, I just told you, don't you remember?" A comment like this is invalidation and a rejection of what she is experiencing. I was judging her by saying, "Do you remember?" Of course she didn't. It caused her to feel ashamed, which was not my intention. I said it because I was impatient.

When I heard Mom saying "she had to go to work and see her patients at the clinic," I knew that she was attempting to be accepted in her unique identity. Maybe she needed to use the toilet but could not express that need. By honoring what she said and asking her to tell me more, she felt understood, loved, and accepted. I answered her by saying, "You sound concerned." This response allowed her to tell me more about her emotional experience.

STEP THREE: SELF-ASSESSMENT TOOL

Do you want to correct, argue, and reason about what the person with Alzheimer's is telling you?

Do you take what he is saying to you personally?

Do you get impatient when he is talking about something that you cannot understand?

Do you feel annoyed with constant repetition of requests?

If you answered yes to any of these questions, validation is a tool to use.

STEP THREE: EXERCISE

Of the four statements above in the self-assessment tool, which would you rate as the number one most difficult situation for you?

Now complete the sentence below using the statement you chose as most difficult .

When a person with Alzheimer's is completely wrong in what they are saying but insists or argues with me I feel _____.

When a person with Alzheimer's is verbally abusive or ugly to me I feel _____.

When a person with Alzheimer's babbles nonsense nonstop I feel _____.

When a person with Alzheimer's asks me the same thing over and over I feel_____.

STEP THREE: BREATHING EXERCISE-

NOTE: As you become familiar with controlled breathing by doing it often, it will become an automatic response and you will not need to read these preliminary directions and can just go forward to the exercise specific to this step.

This mindfulness of your breathing will bring oxygen to your brain, slow your heart rate and give you a frame of mind that is compassionate for your mind and heart.

BEFORE you begin any breathing exercise first pay attention to how you are breathing and what you are feeling at the moment.

Find a quiet place where you can be alone for at least a few moments. It can be outside by a pond or in a bathroom stall at your office. You just don't want to be disturbed.

Close your eyes and begin to breathe in deeply and slowly. Breathe through your nose or mouth, which ever feels most natural to you.

As you inhale, connect with your feeling by clearly naming it. Many times our feelings seem to swirl around us in confusion, especially in emotionally charged situations.

When you name the feeling you are stopping that emotional "overload".

Now that you have named the feeling (love, hurt, compassion, frustration, joy), allow it to expand as the air fills your lungs.

Let the feeling grow larger and larger.

Let it fill you entirely, and as it does allow yourself to focus deeply on the feeling.

Imagine it flowing throughout your body along with the oxygen you are inhaling, and let it travel until it has reached the tips of your fingers, the top of your head, the soles of your feet, and behind your closed eyes.

Now slowly release your breath through your nose or your mouth, whichever is more comfortable.

As you exhale, release the feeling along with your breath.

Feel it slipping out.

Empty your body of it - let it go.

As you do, can you sense the parts of your body that suddenly feel lighter? Less tense? Somehow emptied?

This exercise can work in very powerful ways, whether dealing with positive of negative emotions or even the feeling of being overwhelmed, because all emotions can be stressful until acknowledged and directed.

The **third step breathing exercise** focuses on our goal of using validation in compassionate caring of the person with Alzheimer's. To reinforce that our own emotions can cause us difficulty in successful validation, complete the breathing exercise using the feeling you wrote down from the exercise above.

Now that you have named the emotion, begin the breathing exercise again.

As you do, can you sense the parts of your body that suddenly feel lighter? Less tense? Somehow emptied?

Like the first two steps, we can use the breathing exercise to first recognize and focus on our personal "emotional triggers" and then to defuse their power over our reaction.

Imagine acknowledging the person with Alzheimer's and focusing on his feelings.

Now breathe into the tenderness where you feel your place of compassion. Listen with a tender heart. Feel your heart connecting with his. Imagine sitting patiently and holding onto tenderness. Imagine listening with an open heart, filled with compassion and without any judgment. Judgmental thinking such as "This is good, this is bad, I want out of here" or "What's the matter with him?" creates barriers

Here are some simple phrases that you can use to validate the person when he is trying to communicate to you.

"Tell me more."

"I am curious about what you are saying."

"I hear what you are saying and can imagine how you must feel."

"It sounds like this is important to you."

You can also repeat what he just told you using his own words with the added Aww, Ohh, Mmm,

Any request for a complicated explanation may be too much for him to articulate to you. He may not be aware of his feelings, but the experience he is describing may be a clue.

If he says, "I have to go to work right now; where is my car?" You can respond by saying, "Oh, you have to go to work? Tell me more," and then listen.

Now that you have rehearsed this process in your imagination, practice. Remember that it is about the person's feelings, not about the words.

STEP THREE AFFIRMATIONS:

"I listen with an open heart".

"I connect with what is alive by listening with my entire being."

"I validate the aliveness in this person".

"I create a place of love and safety by how I listen and demonstrate understanding with empathy."

BENEFITS OF STEP THREE

To validate a person with Alzheimer's is to allow him to feel safe, trusted, nurtured, and honored for his unique identity and individuality. It is one more powerful tool to use as you continue to grow as a compassionate caregiver.

Just as with any other skill, practice will both increase your expertise and also encourage you to create your own variations or challenge yourself to go further.

For example, in the step you were only asked to work on the statement that you rated number one as causing greatest difficulty or stress, but there is no reason why you can't go back and work on the statements you identify as concerns, or even write down your own statements.

You are probably picking up that these steps are not only about providing tools for working with the Alzheimer's patient but also steps in self-growth.

The path to guidance is one of love and compassion, not of force and coercion. - Anonnymous

STEP FOUR: COMPASSIONATE DISTRACTION

Distraction, used as a method of commu-nication, provides mental relaxation, amusement, and diversion. Distraction af-ter validation is bringing the person with Alzheimer's to an emotionally safe place. Wherever she thinks she is, that is where she is. We meet her there, using our imagina-tion and capturing her feelings.

Distraction shifts the attention from dis-tress to compassion and comfort for the person.

Distraction is particularly useful when someone is agitated.

As discussed in Step Three, the person with Alzheimer's wants to feel heard and validated.

Step Four is the technique of using dis-traction. It is acknowledging and honoring what the person with Alzheimer is saying or doing and then gently taking her mind off what is troubling her. The mind cannot entertain more than one emotion at the same time. Distraction redirects distressful thinking and feelings.

One effective distraction technique is music. Using music for distracting and redirecting usually guarantees successful diversions. Almost every part of the brain is affected by music, as it produces a universal response and alters mood.

In the late stages of Alzheimer's, language is affected and the person may not be able to understand what you are saying and they often cannot speak well. It has been demonstrated that the patient responds positively to a song or tune.

Sound is associated with long-term memory and feelings, and music affects the deep part of our brain, the limbic system, where feelings are processed. Familiar sounds and songs decrease agitation and are a good way of distracting. Sharing music is a compassionate experience for both the caretaker and the person with Alzheimer's.

" Music expresses that which cannot be put into words and that which cannot remain silent." - Victor Hugo

Try using the suggested techniques below:

❖ Rhythmic, usually repetitive, recitation of words or phrases (i.e. "Three blind mice, three blind mice, see how they run, see how they run....")

❖ Song-like qualities such as words or phrases on one, two, or three notes.

❖ Solo beginnings where one person starts which then spread to the group (i.e. " Row, row , row your boat...").

Early childhood songs are favorites for people with Alzheimer's. You might pick out a known melody such as: "Three Blind Mice" and put new words to it: "One clean shirt, one clean shirt, this is how we dress. First we put it over your head," and so on.

Singing or humming as a form of distraction in a calm tone is comforting. The person with Alzheimer's may have learned songs in childhood such as "Mary Had A Little Lamb," "You Are My Sunshine," "Happy Birthday," and "Row Your Boat," as well as lullabies, carols, and hymns. Many of these songs are deeply ingrained in the mind and associated with happy times. Although the memory may be gone the music is still able to invoke positive emotion.

Knowing early rhyming songs helps the caretaker to connect with the person with Alzheimer's and allows her to connect and participate actively. It is a positive mode of distraction. Have fun doing it! It makes each day of your lives together a little more joyous.

Another way to use distraction as a form of compassion is to direct the person toward something that is calming and meaningful to her. In this case, it is crucial to know the things that she cherishes (such as a photo album) or hobbies she is still interested in. Effective distraction as a form of compassion can come only with time and effort, particularly if you are caring for someone you haven't known for long. You will want to talk to family or friends to elicit ideas.

She may not remember where she is going, where she is, if she needs to go to the toilet, or if she is in pain. She may have lost her language skills and need social interaction to feel connected. She may be tired or be experiencing side effects from a medication. She may be acting out or trying to wander away (or elope).

The caretaker needs to capture the feeling that she is expressing. Validating what she may be acting out and making sure that she is safe, then distraction, is a compassionate form of focusing on her. To effectively distract the patient, find hobbies or activities that are meaningful to her. Stories about family members, jokes, discussing personal "stories" or even a meeting with a social service worker may fill in some blanks. Stay curious and experiment, keep track of what works and what has not. You will find out what works best for her in different situations and add joy to her world.

Tom was a caretaker to a very dear but highly excitable Alzheimer's person. Early on, he learned that she'd had a hidden guilty pleasure throughout her life. She had been an international buyer in the fashion industry, and her role meant that she had to maintain a lifestyle and figure similar to that of a model.

However, she loved sweets so desperately that she confessed she'd sometimes buy a container of icing or ice cream, hide it in her apartment, and eat the entire container in an orgy of chocolate, sometimes just using her fingers as she indulged. This was a lady with a serious sweet tooth!

Eventually, she lost her ability to communicate coherently. When she appeared to be heading toward a blue moment, he started to talk about his favorite flavor of ice cream and more often than not her face would light up. What a delicious way to distract!

LESLIE'S STORY

Leslie was a resident aide who worked at an assisted living facility. She talked to an anxious resident named Irma and tried to distract her by engaging her in a football game on TV and joining in the party. It was the Super Bowl Party, and the Leslie was excited to view it. In fact, she thought everyone in the facility would be excited to watch the extravaganza on the big-screen TV.

Irma had no interest whatsoever in football. The more that Leslie tried to get her to watch the game, the more Irma resisted and insisted that she had to "go to make dinner for her babies."

Leslie then remembered that Irma loved to cook. She asked Irma to help serve popcorn and punch for the Super Bowl party, which was exactly what Irma wanted to do. It was important to Irma that she feel that she was needed and had a purpose.

The key to distraction is not avoidance but using a short-term tool to get through difficult periods. It is helpful to provide alternatives to the person with Alzheimer's. Using distraction, followed by validating feelings, is an effective method for cooperating compassionately and safely.

STEP FOUR: SELF-ASSESSMENT TOOL

❖ Does the person with Alzheimer's become anxious when you try to force her to do something you think is fun?
❖ Does she try to elope or wander?
❖ Does she participate in activities such as clipping coupons, looking at magazine pictures, folding socks or towels, looking at a photo album, singing, humming, dancing, or tapping her feet or hands when you hum?
❖ Does she seem to be looking for someone?
❖ Have you focused only on a task

71

to be accomplished (such as toileting) without also singing or talking about something that is meaningful to her?

If you answered yes to any of these questions, the Step Four exercises may be helpful.

STEP FOUR: EXERCISE

List what unmet needs might be triggering the person's agitation. For example, has she been to the toilet in the last two hours? Have you spoken about her past in the last hour? Is she bored?

List several activities that she currently likes to engage in.

List several activities that she loved to do in the past.

List three or four people, pets, places, and events that she cherished in the past.

List the things you know she does not like to do.

What music does she respond to, especially songs from her early life?

List the environmental sounds or people that might be annoying to her. Might it be confusing when several people are talking at once? Phones ringing? A loud TV or music she does not like? Is she being ignored while others are talking around her? Are there people she does not recognize? (Sadly, my mom did not recognize my husband, David, and kept asking, "Who is he?")

Distraction techniques work best when tailored to knowledge of the individual and their likes and dislikes and personal history.

Can you think of any techniques that would work for the person that you are caring for? Write them here:

_____

_____

_____

It is important to know about these issues before you interact with the person.
Planning ahead prevents anxiety, panic, or
anger. Announce what you are going to do
before you do an activity. Remember that
validation always comes before distraction.
Keep a diary of your efforts, and practice
the distraction techniques or activities that
have been successful.

STEP FOUR: BREATHING EXERCISE-

NOTE: As you become familiar with controlled breathing by doing it often, it will become an automatic response and you will
not need to read these preliminary directions and can just go forward to the exercise specific to this step.

This mindfulness of your breathing will bring
oxygen to your brain, slow your heart rate
and give you a frame of mind that is compassionate for your mind and heart.

BEFORE you begin any breathing exercise
first pay attention to how you are breathing
and what you are feeling at the moment.

Find a quiet place where you can be alone for at least a few moments. It can be outside by a pond or in a bathroom stall at your office. You just don't want to be disturbed.

Close your eyes and begin to breathe in deeply and slowly. Breathe through your nose or mouth, which ever feels most natural to you.

As you inhale connect with your feeling by clearly naming it. Many times our feelings seem to swirl around us in confusion, especially in emotionally charged situations.

When you name the feeling, you are stopping that emotional "overload".

Now that you have named the feeling (love, hurt, compassion, frustration, joy), allow it to expand as the air fills your lungs.

Let the feeling grow larger and larger.

Let it fill you entirely and as it does allow yourself to focus deeply on the feeling.

Imagine it flowing throughout your body along with the oxygen you are inhaling and let it travel until it has reached the tips of your fingers, the top of your head, the soles of your feet, and behind your closed eyes.

Now slowly release your breath through your nose or your mouth whichever is more comfortable.

As you exhale, release the feeling along with your breath.

Feel it slipping out.

Empty your body of it - let it go.

As you do, can you sense the parts of your body that suddenly feel lighter? Less tense? Somehow emptied?

This exercise can work in very powerful ways, whether dealing with positive of negative emotions or even the feeling of being overwhelmed, because all emotions can be stressful until acknowledged and directed.

The **fourth step breathing exercise** focuses on our goal of using distraction in compassionate caregiving. Along with the benefits of adding oxygen to our bloodstream, our thinking becomes more focused, de-stressing emotional overload and increasing awareness of our body. In this step, breathing and focus are joined with the intent of deep relaxation for the caretaker.

The feeling you will use is happiness. As you progress through your breathing and body awareness ask yourself how each part of your body is capable of expressing happiness. Does the tension in your lips and even their shape change? What happens to the edges of your eyes and even with your eyes closed do you seem to be "looking" at something? What is the position of your hands? Are they palm up or down? Are your fists open? Continue this exercise and allow yourself to have some moments of distraction from your hard work.

As you complete the exercise, focus on how you are feeling.

STEP FOUR: AFFIRMATIONS

"I am compassionate and sensitive. I am validating first then distracting to another activity."

STEP FOUR BENEFITS

Distraction takes her mind off something that may be troubling the Alzheimer's patient. She may not even know what is troubling her and may be unable to use words to describe the problem.

Once again you are adding additional tools and techniques to your caretaking repetoire for the Alzheimer's person and have experienced the added value of distraction for yourself.

"Life is easier than you think.

All you have to do is:

Accept the impossible,

Do without the indispensable,

Bear the intolerable, and

Be able to smile at anything." —— Anonymous

STEP FIVE: COMPASSIONATE COMMUNICATION

Communication is a connection between two people. It is sending and receiving messages or information by sound, signals, writing, or behavior.

The key is the connection. We have all watched people participate in what appears to be communication but realize that one of the parties is not part of the communication at all. One may be "sending," but unless the other person is actively "receiving," there is no communication.

Actively listening to another human being is one of the greatest gestures of compassion. It is a form of empathy, because whether or not the other party agrees with what is being communicated, the surety of having been "heard and understood" acknowledges the person's value and is a sincere sign of respect.

I have heard this type of misleading exchange between caretakers and people with Alzheimer's: "Can you hear me?

What's the matter?" The answer given may be, "Yeah, I hear you" or a blank stare.

On average, people remember only 20 percent of what they hear. The remaining 80 percent of communication depends mostly on feeling, perception, and state of mind, not words.

With an Alzheimer's patient, because the speech portion of the brain deteriorates, communication can be challenging. The caregiver who consciously communicates with compassion creates a positive feeling about the exchange for the person. Although the words may not register or he no longer understands the words depending on the stage of the disease, tenderness, safety, acknowledgement, acceptance, respect, and warmth can be conveyed. What a powerful message to send to a person living in what can be a very confusing world—it is a powerful message for anyone with or without Alzheimer's.

Think of the saying "Listen with your heart." People who have opened themselves to that experience, or have been lucky enough to be the recipient of that level of communication, nod and usually smile when they hear the phrase. When I listen with my heart, it is like meditating or praying. The person I care about becomes my entire focus, and I think, "I truly want to hear you. I am not just going to hear your words, I am going to listen to you with all my being. I am making myself quiet to everything else around us, and I am opening up all my senses to you."

Do you find that a powerful message?

We've learned that words are only a small fraction of a conversation. Know that the person with Alzheimer's often does not remember much of what you say. Short-term memory loss is part of the disease, and it worsens over time.

Lorrie, a nurse, told me, "As a nurse, I now know that my words and those of the person with Alzheimer's will be only about 20 percent of effective communication. When I realized this, I thought, 'What a gift!

Now I can stop the energy drain and start developing and refining the techniques of the other 80 percent. Being aware of this allowed me to focus on what was effective for the person with the disease."

Our goal as caretakers is effective, compassionate communication that comes from that tender place in the heart. When you think about care, love, and compassion, where do you feel them in your mind and body? Shut your eyes for a moment and locate those places.

Consider your reaction to these phrases:

"Heart-felt laughter" (Do you feel it in your gut or somewhere else in your body?)

"Have a heart" (Do you feel it in your hands or somewhere else in your body?)

"Laughing heartily" (Do you feel this in your lungs or somewhere else in your body?)

"Heart felt moments" (Do you feel this behind your eyes or somewhere else in your body?)

"With all my heart

"Hungry heart"

"Like my heart was going to burst with joy"

"Heart in hand"

"Get to the heart of the matter"

"It broke my heart!"

As you listen with your entire being, as you've just done with this exercise, you sensitize yourself to two things: your unique receptors to emotion and communication and the many ways that you can "hear" without using your ears. How can you use that skill to "hear" what the person with Alzheimer's is trying to communicate with you beyond the measly 20 percent of words?

We just looked at how many parts of our own body the "heart" is in. When we see the closed eyes, tensed hands, quick breathing, clenched gut, or restless feet of the person we are caring for, what might he be trying to communicate to us?

By being attentive, the person with Alzheimer's will receive the signal that you are approachable, genuine, and trustworthy as he attempts to communicate. He will relax and be more receptive to your communication, because you are able to use different channels to send and receive messages.

For the Alzheimer's patient, you are a mirror that helps him to understand time, place, and person. This means that he is watching your face, how fast you move, your eyes, the tone of your voice, and how you are touching him, and he will react to all these messages. As you communicate with him, use your skills to create positive and compassionate communication.

Perhaps you can identify with the following scenario. John went to a doctor's office for a consultation and told me this story. "I spent my time reading a book in the examination room, waiting for the doctor to appear. Suddenly the door flung open, and the doctor came in. I jumped and could feel my heart pounding. I was angry at the disrespect shown to me. I realized that my own doctor quietly tapped on the door before entering. In fact, I think she makes a bit of noise in the hallway even before tapping."

Have you come across people who speak before they have your attention and half of what they need to tell you is lost? Or they talk with their back to you? They often become annoyed when you respond with "What did you say?"

Many people develop hearing problems as they get older. People who work with the hearing impaired suggest gently touching the person's hand or arm to gain his attention before speaking.

STEP FIVE: SELF-AWARENESS TOOL

❖ Do you knock, wave, and
   introduce yourself when
   approaching the person with
   Alzheimer's?
❖ Are you aware of the noise you
   make and the sound level of
   your voice?
❖ Do you use physical cues to signal
   that you are friendly (your
   smile, gentle hand gestures)?
❖ Do you move slowly?
❖ Does your tone of voice convey
   calmness?
❖ Do you sit or squat next to him
   rather than stand over him?
❖ If you answered yes to more than
   one of these questions, try the
   Step Five exercise.

STEP FIVE BREATHING EXERCISE:

The step five breathing exercise is a variation on the breathing exercises we've done
so far. By now you probably have the basic
technique down so that you are easily able
to go through the steps. In step five you are

using your breathing but added along with your own body awareness in your visualization of a caretaking scenario.

Close your eyes. Take an inhalation breath and count from one to four to the bottom of your spine. As you breathe out, part your lips and create a gentle smile.

Imagine that you are approaching the person with Alzheimer's.

Imagine signaling to him when you are ten feet away. It can be a wave or a knock on the door.

When you are five feet away, address him by his proper name (Mrs. Jones, Ms. Sarah, my wonderful Mom Elena).

Introduce yourself each time you approach.

If he does not recognize you, get a photo of yourself and say, "Hi Dad, this is Maria, your daughter."

Avoid using the terms honey, mama, darling, baby, sweetie and other endearments.

They can be perceived as condescending. They are inappropriately intimate and disrespectful to most people, and the person with Alzheimer's is no different. Caretakers in facilities often use these terms, and when asked why, they say it is an endearment. A compassionate greeting includes the person's name unless asked to do otherwise.

Approach him from a diagonal angle; avoid approaching head on or from the back.

Avoid standing over him. This posture can be interpreted as aggressive and intimidating. Get to eye level. If he is sitting in a chair, pull up a chair or squat and smile.

Face him, look him directly in the eyes, and smile.

Breathe.

Now:

Use your technique of validation and validate something about what the person is saying or doing.

Capture the feeling.

Reach out and ask him to hold your hand, or if his hands are open, hold his hand. Always be aware of the pressure your place on anyone's hands. He may be suffering from arthritis or other issues that can cause even a gentle handshake to be anything but welcome.

"Shake hands with Alzheimer's."

Touch the palm of his hand with yours with his hand over yours. This is a major therapeutic touch point. Palm to palm, allow for the connection and breathe again.

Avoid launching your agenda on him. Wait a few seconds to validate something about this person and then begin to speak about the activities of the day such as breakfast or showering. Remember to validate and connect with him before you begin.

Speak slowly in a moderate voice tone, allowing them to read your lips and see your face well.

If the person wears a hearing aide or glasses make sure both are on.

State one sentence at a time, and use no more than four words in a sentence.

Wait for a response, while looking into his eyes, and smile.

Give no more than two simple choices. For example, you might ask, "Do you want to wear the blue pants or the beige pants?" Stop and wait for his response.

Use gentle hand gestures to help convey your message. Wait for a response.

If he gets agitated, give him a few moments of quiet time and space. It may help to leave the room (if he is safe) so that he can quiet himself.

As he rests walk away from the room and finish your breathing with three deep breaths and open your eyes.

BONUS EXERCISE: HUMOR!!

HUMOR (OR "GOD GIVE ME PATIENCE AND I WANT IT NOW!")

Alzheimer's is no laughing matter, but laughter can help both you and the person with Alzheimer's cope and communicate while alleviating a stressful situation.

The humor is not meant to belittle or cause any negative feelings to persons with Alzheimer's or their caregivers. Laughter and humor are often some of the few things you can share; they help to maintain dignity and communicate light-hearted joy. Laughter relieves stress and sends a non-threatening signal of camaraderie. It can liberate a person from fear, sadness, confusion and even pain. It assures the person with Alzheimer's that everything is all right. When you can seize the opportunity for laughing, it shows that you are present in the moment together. If something even remotely funny happens, laugh!

Those of us who have taken care of a person with Alzheimer's know that hearing aids, dentures, glasses, and the most personal of items get lost frequently and can later turn up in the most unusual places.

I was once told a story about a gentleman who lived in an assisted living facility in Sun City Center, Florida. He complained to another resident, "I just bought another hearing aid. I am going broke buying dentures and replacing the hearing aids that I lose. This one cost me four thousand dollars, and it is state of the art —the best I ever had."

"Really?" The neighbor asked, "what kind is it?"

"Twelve thirty," he said.

Other residents nearby started a belly roll laugh, and suddenly everyone around was laughing out loud.

I often hear that "Life is often disguised as humor." I believe that there is truth to that concept and try to evoke laughter as often as I can.

I hear all types of caretakers—attorneys, law enforcement, bankers, doctors and facility administrators—in my workshops saying, "We do not have time to do this." I assure you that using these techniques will take less time and allow everyone to feel the rewards of compassionate communication.

At one of my workshops, we compared volunteer caretakers who have used compassionate, validating, and distraction communicating techniques with those who were task driven. I found through informal interviews that it takes far less time and is far more rewarding to set the stage for communication rather than bossing people into activities. Being bossy does not pay off. The person with Alzheimer's will fight back because he is feeling controlled, resistant, and upset. He feels he is being pushed around, leaving the caretaker dealing with an agitated person. As a result, even more behavioral issues may emerge, lingering for some time and transferring to others. There is a cascading effect for everyone.

Realistically, we all know a caretaker has limited time and much to accomplish. However, launching into an agenda with the person right away will create resistance.

Take the few seconds to experiment with the techniques discussed. Validate the individual and connect with him before "time to get up, time for breakfast, time for a shower," etc.

See which techniques work best for you and for the person you are caring for and then build your own repertoire. Not all of the techniques will work every time or with every person, so you need to keep adding to your toolbox. Otherwise, you'll demonstrate the idea that "if the only tool you own is a hammer, you'll treat every problem as though it is a nail."

Avoid physically crowding the person with Alzheimer's. If he is agitated, bringing another person in to help often increases the agitation, because it may feel like he is being cornered. When a person feels like he is losing control, he reverts to the "fight or flight" response. This is our survival mechanism when feeling threatened.

Use the tools you have been collecting—if one technique doesn't work, put down "the hammer" and reach for another technique. Is this a moment to softly sing? Perhaps this singing is a time to invoke a memory. Is it a time when humor can be used and shared?

Zora, the co-author of this book, told me of one of those "Aha" moments we hear about when she was caring for her dad.

"When my dad moved cross country to live with us, it was a hard adjustment for everyone, despite all best intentions. He lost his independence along with his driver's license, his house, his friends, and many activities that he enjoyed. In addition to his decline in functioning, being severely hearing impaired limited our ability to keep him entertained, and he got bored easily.
One night, my husband turned on the TV to watch the movie The Lord of the Rings. I fully expected my dad, a retired mechanical engineer, to complain about how silly it was. I was totally surprised when I looked over to see that not only was he not fidgeting

but he was sitting forward, smiling, and utterly transfixed by the movie. My father had discovered the magic of animated movies! Every once in a while, he'd say, 'Noooo' in a wondering voice."

"What a wonderful evening we had sharing that evening. We were all laughing. Afterward, he kept asking, 'Where did they find such people? Did you see what that little skinny one did?' He truly believed that the places and characters were real. For my husband and I, we'd found a way to share many happy hours together with Dad.

"At another time, my very proper father giggled through Shrek! He and my husband cheerfully settled down to nights of Star Wars, and I was shushed if I interrupted. I rarely did.

"Although my Dad is gone now, the laughter we shared those nights still brings a smile."

ELSA'S STORY-

Another story about humor came from Elsa. "My mother sees people in her room that are not there. I walked into her room one time, and it was torn apart; there were sheets everywhere.. I reacted by nearly screaming at her, telling her there were no people in the room and quickly trying to straighten out the room."

When Elsa got upset, it only upset her mother more. Feeling hopelessness, Elsa began to cry, and her mother started crying too. They both were standing on a heap of sheets.

Elsa then realized that in the midst of the chaos, she and her mother were actually sharing a powerful experience.

She started laughing. There Elsa was sitting in a heap of sheets, feeling out of control and powerless, with her mother who also was sitting in a heap of sheets and feeling the same way. Elsa's ability to detach and laugh caused her mother to stop and laugh as well. The situation turned from panic and distress to laughter.

Elsa said, "Laughing was all I could do, because I saw that my tears only made Mom's situation worse. I was powerless, but I could also see my situation and feel great compassion toward Mom, who was helpless and losing her mind to Alzheimer's disease. I also felt my mother's compassion for me as she put her arms around me, held my hand and comforted me, and looked into my eyes. It was a moment when we held each other in love. For me it was a feeling, an understanding that we both were powerless yet able to share love. My fear of losing control dissipated with the laughter, and the fear that Mom felt also dissipated with laughter. All that is real is the present moment. Mom taught me that."

Hearing Elsa's story, I am reminded of the songs, movies, poems, and times in my life when there was laughter through tears.

If I asked a room full of caretakers whether they could relate to Elsa's story, I suspect that most would say yes.

STEP FIVE: AFFIRMATIONS

"My smile communicates compassion."

"My eyes communicate kindness."

"My touch communicates care."

"My body language communicates safety and approachability."

STEP FIVE: BENEFITS

Awareness of how to communicate effectively and with compassion is a win-win solution for all interactions with Alzheimer's patients. You will find the person responsive to your approach when using these techniques. You will feel proactive and be able to support him in his activities of daily life.

In Step Five we've discussed the therapeutic uses of humor in caretaking and as part of making a connection with the person with Alzheimer's.

We've also used a variation on breathing exercises that is a technique we might want to call active practice.

It is lack of love for ourselves that inhibits our compassion toward others. If we make friends with ourselves, there is no obstacle to opening our hearts and minds to others. — Anonymous

When you come to the edge of all that you know, you must believe two things: there will be air to breathe, and you will be given wings to fly. — Anonymous

STEP SIX: COMPASSION TOWARD SELF

Compassion toward self means meeting your needs for your well-being. Let's call this self-empathy. A key part of living compassionately is giving loving attention to yourself.

Insightful caretakers recognize that they have the power to change their relation to the present moment by using on themselves the same compassionate tools they provide to others.

This is critical because caregivers are at high risk for break down. About fifteen million people provide care for people with Alzheimer's. At least 75 percent of their visits to primary care physicians are stress related, and approximately 65 percent of all caregivers die before the person with Alzheimer's dies. Suicide and homicide rates are higher among caretakers of Alzheimer's family members. Divorce rates are higher, and caretakers are at risk for drug and alcohol abuse.

Shawn, a caregiver, told me, "My brother-in-law, Jim, died care taking his father. He took his father's morphine and overdosed in the room next to him."

My friend, Sierra, told me how she took her mother's fentanyl transdermal pain medication patch and ended up in the emergency room with serious side effects. When I asked her why she did this, she said, "I just wanted to be numb and escape for a few minutes. Taking care of my dad, who has been struggling with Alzheimer's for nine years, burnt me out."

Balance is the key to physical and emotional well-being. Being compassionate to yourself brings clarity, a positive perspective, and self-knowledge. It is being proactive rather than reactive. We have all heard the saying that you cannot love someone else if you do not love yourself. Loving yourself is letting go of judgment and negative self-evaluation. It prevents "spiritual indigestion."

In my job, I travel a great deal, so I'm on and off airplanes constantly, and each time I fly, I get a useful reminder about being a caretaker.

At the start of each flight, the attendant instructs the passengers about safety issues. The first instruction is that if the oxygen mask drops, you need to put it on yourself before you try to put one on anyone else. This reminds me that I can't take care of anyone else until I take care of myself.

The second instruction is to remain seated and keep your seatbelt fastened. This reminds me that caretaking is a "bumpy ride", and that being strapped in will help me maintain balance when things get rough.

Then I hear the flight attendant's advice about using the seat cushion as a floatation device should the plane crash in the ocean. I remember that if we consciously use our caretaking skills with ourselves, we can stay afloat in a turbulent world.

A caregiver by the name of Conrada told me that she'd realized that she needed to use self-care tools instead of thinking there would be "time later." She said, "If not me, who? If I get sick and am unable to do anything because I am so stressed, who will take care of me and my Mom?" This was a terrifying thought for us both!"

We'd all agree that treating yourself poorly makes no sense, yet caregivers often fail to seek help. Why? Some of the following reasons are commonly mentioned:

They are in denial about their own mental and physical care issues.

They minimize their symptoms, telling themselves that they are not as bad off as the person with Alzheimer's.

They tell themselves that they don't have time right now to take care of themselves.

They are overwhelmed.

They feel guilty or disloyal about complaining.

They fear what will happen to the Alzheimer's patient if they are not there to care for her.

Can you think of others?

All caregivers experience stress, especially if they are task driven. The hormone cortisol is released in the body during times of stress. It increases your blood pressure, heart rate, and muscle tension. It affects the immune system and promotes wear and tear on the body.

Our thoughts affect brain chemistry, and negative thinking creates negative responses in the body. This response is similar to an animal's survival instinct. As mentioned earlier, when we feel stress, we respond with a "flight or flight" response. Imagine that a ferocious, hungry tiger is running toward you. You can run or fight—the choice is simple!

Today we know that unlike the spike of hormones in those unpleasant moments of sudden stress, the "quiet" everyday stress that caregivers feel is much more dangerous. Think of it this way. There is the tiger again, and you make a decision. The hormones go wild, peak, and stop (especially if you made the wrong choice—oops, but the situation is resolved).

As a caregiver, you have a "tiger" sitting close to you each time you interact with the person with Alzheimer's. You know it is there, and you know that you have no choice but to take your chances on that path. You think about what might happen over and over, day after day. The cortisol keeps flowing, because the stress response never ends. The issue never resolves. You exhaust yourself and use up your reserves.

When your thoughts are pessimistic and negative, your body responds as though you need to run or fight. When the situation is chronic, your body breaks down. If you are driven by fear and anxiety, you overstimulate the brain to the point of burnout.

That same part of the brain responds to how you talk to yourself and your interpretation of your experience as a caretaker. Your experiences are what you say about them, as you are what you think. The only way to change negative self-talk is through compassion, talking to yourself positively and avoiding judgment.

Positive self-talk is using kind words rather than talking to yourself like a bossy bully. Let go of an inner dialogue of should, have to, always, never, got to, and must. These words guarantee a negative response in the body.

No one likes to be told what to do. This is a losing battle, and the person who talks to herself negatively is the loser.

Sonya, another caretaker, told me, "I always put my mother first. I tormented myself in my negative self-talk. I could barely get through the day, and I was lucky to sneak in a shower and brush my own teeth."

I hear similar stories constantly from caretakers. Caring for the person with Alzheimer's is exhausting and stressful. Tasks become overwhelming, and if they are the focus, they become shallow experiences with no reward.

Living in a world of negative self-talk destroys compassion. It makes life cold and robotic, creates resentment, and sets us up to feel like victims. There is no sense of personal choice or ownership of our emotional well-being.

Frank, a client of mine, told me, "I am always just in reaction mode and a reactive state of mind. I have a constant stream of thoughts, even in my sleep. I wake up drenched in sweat and with sore shoulders as if I were digging a ditch all night. One morning I woke up with chest pain and shortness of breath, I was rushed to the emergency room, and found that I was having a heart attack."

A caretaker named Cary said, "I cannot take time for myself, I feel like I am complaining all the time, and I hate complainers. I don't want to be like that. The last thing I want is to be thought of as a victim. I do not want anyone to feel sorry for me."

These testimonials speak to the wear and tear of caregiving.

Broadening our experience by being in touch with our feelings starts with self-talk, and positive words allow us to respond with positive thought and deeds.

In my Compassionate Communication Training Program, we play a game called My Inner Dialogue. We discuss how we can think of a task as an "I choose to" or as an "I have to."

We list tasks and assign "I chose to" or "I have to" phrases to them. We decide which feels better and which gives a sense of empowerment.

Here is an example. Colleen, a caretaker, said: "If I choose to help Mom with a shower, I own the experience. If my self-talk is 'I have to,' it feels like I am being commanded to do so, and I feel resentful, even though it's me telling myself these things."

Negative self-talk creates even more negative self-talk, and with each task, we feel more stress. It's called "dumping on yourself, " and it is no wonder that caretakers feel exhausted.

Another client of mine, David, told me, "I started being aware of my choices in how I talk to myself. When I do this, it brings me back to the basics of asking myself, what is my intention? My self-talk changes from a should, must, or got to to more empowering words: I want to, I choose to, I prefer to, I am happy to! I notice that my feelings follow, and my mind and heart begin to soften."

I was told once about oxytocin, which is sometimes called the "love hormone." The release of this hormone and other feelgood, opiate-like chemicals is related to states of trust and empathy. They have positive physiological effects on our bodies.

Negative thinking = negative response!

Compassionate thinking = positive response!

We can enhance compassion just by thinking about kindness, compassion, patience, and tolerance, and of course by breathing fully. When I do this, I can feel physical changes within eight seconds. I notice my body letting go of the tension that I hold in my shoulders, as though I were letting go of the weight of the world.

Releasing negative self-talk and choosing to use kind words are part of the balancing act of being compassionate and making healthy choices. There is a relationship between negative self-talk and how we care for ourselves. If we are having a negative dialogue with ourselves, there is a good chance our self care is also negative and neglectful.

When my self-talk was negative, I might have said, "I had no time to exercise, no time to stretch out on the yoga mat, no time to eat fresh food, no time to pray and meditate. I have to do more and get as much done as I can cram into a day." By saying "I have no time" I closed off from things that were nurturing. I did not want to talk to my family or friends, and I began to isolate. I stopped caring for myself. I ate junk food, gained weight, felt horrid, and tried to zone out by watching mindless TV. My body could not escape. It was holding on to stress, and I felt terribly unhealthy and distressed.

My mind circled around and around, and I obsessed about what I needed to do even when I'd completed the tasks I'd assigned myself. I woke up exhausted and spent the days wishing they would come to an end.

If I did something for myself, I was not "taking care of Mom and doing everything for her." It was a trap of guilt that I'd built for myself.

Does this sound familiar?

STEP SIX: SELF-ASSESSMENT TOOL

❖ Are you providing caretaking
but no self-care? Or do you
consciously practice self-care

by drinking water, exercising,
eating fresh fruits and
vegetables, doing breathing
exercises, calling friends, and
praying or meditating?
❖ Can you stop worrying?
❖ Are you restless and on edge?
❖ Do you experience muscle
pain in your neck and back,
headache, or stomach
problems?
❖ Are you using junk food, drugs,
alcohol, or gambling to
escape stress?

If you answered yes to any of the above, you are choosing self-negligence rather than self-compassion. This means that you are choosing to ignore yourself.

Morgan told me that he keeps an "A to Z inventory of gratitude." At the end of each day, he reminds himself of what he has done well, how he was compassionate, and the little things that he experienced throughout the day. He might start with A for apple. "I took a bite of a tart green apple and noticed how my mouth burst with a reaction. I felt alive! I thought of how Mom lost her sensation of taste, but I still had mine. I savored the experience. Then I noticed that crunching felt good—again, Mom could no longer do this or swallow well. I felt gratitude for what I had and empathy for Mom's loss of her sense of taste. I then took Mom out to the zoo. We went all over looking at the animals and though I was pushing her in her wheelchair, we had almost child-like wonder at the experience of being at the zoo together. It's the little big things that I became so grateful for."

What a wonderful way to celebrate the day's treasures!

Try this exercise. Shut your eyes as though you are ready to go to sleep after a hard day of caretaking. Think of these messages:

"I didn't get half of what needed to done."

"The house is a mess."

"Mom was so fretful and anxious all day."

"I feel so tired and guilty and angry, and tomorrow is just more of the same."

"I feel so hopeless."

Do you feel tension in your body? Do you think you will sleep well if you sleep at all?

Let's try again. Shut your eyes and take a few slow, deep breaths. Think of these messages:

"I decided to stop trying to clean the house and chose to comfort Mom today."

"I didn't realize how dry her hands had become. Massaging them with lotion felt so good to both of us."

How does your body feel now? Do you think you might get some well-deserved and much-needed rest?

As we recognize that we can change our relation to the present moment by being compassionate to ourselves, we empower ourselves.

Being in a state of gratitude is one way of being compassionate to ourselves.

Try Morgan's "A to Z gratitude list." It is guaranteed to reduce negativity and increase your awareness of how the "little big things" in your life are a blessing.

Being compassionate to yourself allows you to get perspective, clarity, and wisdom. It is choosing stress management and ease versus dis-ease.

STEP SIX: EXERCISE

1. How many hours per day do you spend caretaking, either directly or indirectly (filling out medical forms, running errands, etc.)?
2. How many hours per week do you spend exercising?
3. How many hours per week do you spend praying, meditating, or reflecting on things that you are grateful for?

4. How many fresh fruits and vegetables do you eat each day?
5. How many glasses of water or decaffeinated beverages do you drink each day?
6. How many hours per week do you spend involved in a hobby or other healthy, pleasurable activity (including a support group)?
7. How many hours per night do you sleep?

Rate yourself on a scale of 0 (which is none) to 10 (which is excellent self care) on how much attention you pay to these seven wellness steps.

When you look at your answers, does it seem like you are balanced in all the categories? If you were a tire on say a car, would the ride be smooth or bumpy?

If we give "everything" in one category and "nothing" in another, we are unbalanced.

STEP SIX: BREATHING EXERCISE

The **step six breathing exercise** is another variation on the breathing exercises we've done so far. By now you probably have the basic technique down so that you are easily able to go through the step. This exercise is great to use when you really need to calm down.

Focus on building your inner strength. Try this breathing technique.

As you inhale, think, "The strength I feel inside me is enough to sustain me during any experience I have today.

As you exhale, say to yourself, "The compassion from my heart will lead me in helping (him or her)."

With such thoughts, we bring compassion into our lives, which helps us become strong and compassionate toward others.

Relax and allow for rest! Lie down and mentally go over the parts of your body one by one for fifteen to twenty minutes. This exercise has some great payoffs. You slow down your racing thoughts. Your train your mind to concentrate on the parts of your body instead of all the "things" that you "should" be thinking about or doing.

Your self-dialogue will probably go something like:

Okay, my body parts.

This is so silly.

I don't have time for this.

I'm twitchy, itchy, and this is a waste of my time.

Okay, body part. Arm, yep there it is. Arm is attached. Good job.

Next, mouth.

Wow, my mouth feels so tight. I am going to end up with some major witchy wrinkles.

Okay, big open, close, smile, yawn, wiggle that jaw.

Loosen up old mouth. Come on mouth, big smile, big kiss. Love you.

While doing this exercise, you not only paid lots of very good attention to yourself but you probably giggled a little, felt that you indulged in some self-care, and were able to tune in to your wonderfully unique body.

This is the time when you choose to pay attention to your body. You learn where you uniquely experience body tension. (It might not be your head or stomach—it might be your inability to stop tapping your toe.) You learn to listen to your body and clue in to other things that might be going on in your body. Perhaps that lovable, cushy "muffin top" is a clue that you need to pay more attention to nutrition or to "comfort food" indulgences. Do you hurt somewhere that you have been too busy to acknowledge? This includes your heart, both literally and figuratively.

The payoff has to do with mind, body and spirit. This is your time to slow down and connect with your spiritual side. Have a talk with a part of yourself, thank yourself, and open yourself up to something, whatever floats your spiritual boat.

Remember the floatation cushion? As you review your body parts, take a moment to see how your boat is doing in the stormy seas you travel through life as a caretaker. Is it time to grab your floatation cushion to help you tread water? Do you need a life preserver to help keep your head above water? Or is your boat going down and you need flares and a lifeboat ASAP?

STEP SIX: AFFIRMATIONS

"I give myself permission to be compassionate to myself."

"Being compassionate to myself allows me to keep things in balance."

"Showing Compassion to myself is honoring my life and blessings."

"I eat fresh food and drink water because they are healthy for me and nurture me."

"I meditate or pray to maintain my spiritual connection to the god of my understanding."

"I have an attitude of gratitude, and I list what I am grateful for from A to Z."

BENEFITS OF STEP SIX

Taking care of yourself allows you to see your life in perspective. Just like a wheel, balance is the key. If all parts are not equal, the wheel will not function. If you are balanced mentally, physically, and spiritually, you can be a wise and compassionate caregiver.

One of the most difficult things to give away is kindness; it usually comes back to you.

"We cannot live by ourselves. A thousand threads connect us with each other."

POSITIVE THINKING = POSITIVE RESULTS

NEGATIVE THINKING = NEGATIVE RESULTS

In every book there are choices that need to be made when it comes to progressing through material. When to place self care and compassion in the steps is a hard choice because for caretakers they have often put their own needs aside for so long if we started the book with step six it would seem selfish and self-indulgent to them.

Hopefully the reader has recognized by this point that this book has a double message of compassionate caring. One is for the person who suffers from the brutal effects of Alzheimer's disease, the other is for the caretaker who often bears the brunt of the disease with too little support and too much responsibility.

"*Hope sees the invisible, feels the intangible and achieves the impossible.*" *Anonymous*

"*Don't let what you can't do interfere with what you can do.*" *Anonymous*

"*A lot of us would like to move mountains, but few of us are willing to practice on small hills.*" *Anonymous*

STEP SEVEN: ALLOW OTHERS TO BE COMPASSIONATE

As a caretaker, thinking that you can do it all is setting yourself up for disaster. There is no way to take care of the person with Alzheimer's all by yourself and stay balanced, healthy, and compassionate.

When we first hear the diagnosis of Alzheimer's, it is normal to go into denial. I know I did. Allowing others to support you by sharing their knowledge about end-of-life directives, hospice, and respite care is allowing others to be compassionate. Suffering, disease, chronic illness, and death are difficult and often painful topics of conversation, yet they are necessary.

Upon hearing the diagnosis of Alzheimer's, typical responses include "She is not that bad" or "It might be the stress of Dad's death; she is just lonely." When you make excuses, you may be wondering if you are making something out of nothing.

Facing a disease such as Alzheimer's requires great courage. That is often the situation with elderly couples who have come to depend on each other, as in the following story.

Anna and Wally were neighbors who had become dear friends over the years. Neither had family nearby, and they had supported each other through the loss of their respective spouses. Wally helped Anna with her home maintenance; she fussed at him about getting a haircut. They usually shared at least one meal a day together and enjoyed playing bridge together.

Anna began falling down. The first time it happened, they were taking a morning walk together, and Wally helped to break her fall. The second time, she was alone at home and she broke her arm.

Suddenly, almost at age ninety, Wally became a caretaker. Anna needed help dressing because she couldn't use her arm. She couldn't lift things, and driving was difficult. She was not recovering as quickly as she should.

Her mood swings were initially put down to being depressed about losing her independence. In reality, Anna had Alzheimer's, and she was declining quickly. Within a few months, she was having hallucinations, would wander away from her home, and several times left food cooking on the stove and forgot about it.

Wally began sleeping on the couch in her living room to try to keep her safe from herself, but she fell again and was taken to an emergency room. Luckily for Anna, the hospital staff contacted adult protective services, and she was placed in an Alzheimer's assisted living community.

Wally was in total denial about Anna's diagnosis or his inability to care for her. He lost a good deal of weight and was very depressed, and within a year, he developed serious physical and mental health issues.

In situations like this, asking for help shows courage.

I used to consider asking for help a flaw, a sign of mental and physical weakness. When I first moved to Florida, I was determined to do everything for my mom. I began feeling isolated, disconnected, separate, fragmented, and totally incompetent. There were days when I felt like I was falling apart, which was terrifying—who would take care of Mom if I couldn't?

My mother insisted that she stay at her own home and wanted me with her. She did not want anyone but me in her house taking care of her. I became her nurse, her therapist, her medical secretary, her cook, and her maid, and I did it all with a deluded self-concept of being superwoman or perhaps a super-daughter.

I quickly realized that trying to do everything myself was ego-based. It came from a deep fear that I was not competent or good enough if I could not do everything. When I related this to my best friend, she laughed and said, "Oh really? So you are God now?"

A neighbor saw an ad in a church newsletter, advertising the services of someone who might be able to help me with Mom. I contacted the woman, Lina, and hired her but—no surprise—Mom immediately rejected her.

Lina was an angel in disguise. She was clear about her intentions and told me that she would provide safety and kindness for Mom.

Mom thought of herself as the queen, and said so, and decided that Lina was her servant. Lina did not take this personally. She smiled and found endearing ways to validate Mom. She spoke to Mom gently at eye level, moved slowly, got out of the way when needed, sometimes backing off and going into another room to give Mom space when she "threw a hissy fit." She did not try to control Mom, despite Mom's mean and haughty attitude toward her. On those days that nothing worked for Mom, Lina's sense of humor allowed her to let things roll off her back. While I cringed at my mother's behavior, I marveled at Lina's resilience and began learning from her.

Mom eventually grew to anticipate Lina's arrival and asked for her when she wasn't around. Honesty, I think she enjoyed being with Lina more than being with me. Lina played games with Mom and had her on a predictable routine, and Mom's days went lovingly and smoothly.

Getting Lina's help freed up a few hours, and I joined a support group—in fact, I joined several! (Such was my state of mind by the time Lina arrived to save the day.) I maintained contact with other caretakers and built connections that supported my own well-being.

I was not alone. I was not going insane. I realized it I was safe to express my anger, guilt, sadness, and grief and then laugh at the odd things that no one other than an Alzheimer's caretaker would understand.

The need for support, the level needed, and the ability to obtain support vary.

Zora's experience was different from mine.

"When my dad came to live with me, I thought I was fairly knowledgeable about services, because my entire career had been spent in that arena. I contacted the local elder care agency and told them I needed guidance. I'd never dealt with geriatric issues before, and so I knew nothing about Medicare, transferring insurance, legal issues, etc.

I was extremely lucky to connect with a young woman who helped guide me through the paperwork, and she insisted that my dad have a geriatric specialist as his primary care physician. I'd already contacted my own doctor and would have preferred that he see that physician, but the facility didn't take his insurance.

My dad was born in Europe, and he was old fashioned to the nth degree. In his nineties, he still wore a jacket and tie. He expected to be treated with deference. To top this off, he was almost totally deaf. I'd seen him in action and knew that he would nod and pretend that he understood everything someone told him but walk away having no knowledge at all of what was said.

While complaining that he didn't need to see a doctor, my dad and I went for our initial meeting with Dr. W., a physician who specializes in geriatrics. When I met the doctor, I groaned inwardly. He was so young. However, that was the last time I felt any discomfort with him or his staff.

Dr. W. gently shook my father's hand and said how glad he was to meet him. He maintained eye contact and spoke slowly and clearly, and I could see that my dad was reading his lips. He complimented my dad on his vest and his matching tie and pocket handkerchief and told him that it was nice to see someone who was proud of how he looked. He then took Dad by the arm as though they were good buddies and walked him around the office, introducing him to his staff members, who all stopped, smiled, and said hello. Dad was also assigned a nurse that he was told would normally meet with him.

Dad was glowing and ready to have an exam.

The doctor also asked my Dad's permission if I came in briefly just to help fill out forms.

The doctor spent a long time getting as much history as possible from my dad and I, and he said he'd have all Dad's records sent to him before his next appointment. He also reviewed Dad's medications and asked me about any problems I'd noticed, any concerns I had, and about our home life, exercise, nutrition, interests, friends, and life changes.

He also asked about how things were going for me as a caretaker and urged me to complete a medical power of attorney and an advanced directive. He wasn't morbid, but wasn't shy to address these issues.

Even though my dad couldn't hear the conversation, Dr. W. made a point of asking him questions to keep him involved. He also made the most silly and outrageously awful jokes!

He asked me to step out of the room for the more intimate parts of the exam but made sure that Dad knew I'd be right back. He also said that he would give me all the information so that I could go over it with him.

By the time we left, Dad was grousing about how much the Dr. talked but was eager to hear what he'd said, and I could tell that he was secretly pleased.

Here is what the doctor accomplished in that first visit.

He completely engaged with my dad as an adult and with pride and dignity.

When it appeared that he was simply showing my Dad around, he used the time to begin an evaluation. The gentle handshake checked for arthritis and grip. Walking him around the office checked balance and gait. Talking with eye contact checked hearing and communication, and joking and questions checked Dad's mental acuity.

The doctor made a point of fully involving me as a caretaker while maintaining Dad's integrity. He was concerned about the impact of my dad moving into my home and what support systems were available. He was clear and open in addressing difficult issues, which opened up the lines of communication.

My dad saw Dr. W. many times in the coming years, and he was never kept waiting more than a few minutes, even when he needed to be worked into the schedule. He was always greeted by name and treated graciously and humanely. At the start of each visit, Dr. W. invariably walked into the room and shook Dad's hand, asked him how his card playing was going, complimented him on his attire, and asked me how I was doing.

A few days after my Dad died, I received a phone call from Dr. W., expressing his sympathy and saying how much he would miss my dad. He asked how I was doing, told me what good care my dad had received, and noted how lucky Dad had been to live with me.

Of all the loving calls I received, Dr. W.'s message meant the most to me."

Locating a physician who specializes in geriatric care is critical to addressing all levels of the person's functioning. Geriatric specialists are trained in Alzheimer's issues as well as other elder care issues. They are not perplexed with the multitude of patient needs and are especially able to address the behavioral and safety issues. Additionally, they are part of the support system that the caregiver needs. They can give clear advice regarding what to expect, realistic intervention, and medical/legal issues to consider, and they can check in with caretakers about their own well-being.

Dr. W.'s extended help included advising me that it was time to meet with an attorney and make sure that I could help my dad with upcoming legal issues. When the doctor mentioned this, I lost my breath for a moment, but I was glad that he didn't ignore an issue that he knew would be devastating to my dad if not addressed. By then I knew that I would be calling an attorney who was certified in elder law.

Seeking out this type of medical professional is well worth the effort to both the patient and the caretaker. Even if the person with Alzheimer's is living in a care facility, it is important to check that staff members are trained to deal with the specific issues of this disease.

It may be challenging to address end-of-life issues such advanced directives (a Do Not Resuscitate or DNR, power of attorney, and guardianship if the person with Alzheimer's loses cognitive abilities, and so on), but the issues should not be avoided. In the early stages of the disease, it is helpful to know which resources are available such as hospice, respite or relief care, and social workers. To prevent the reactive crisis management that can occur when the patient starts to decline and cannot participate, these important conversations show your compassion."

STEP SEVEN: SELF-ASSESSMENT TOOL

❖ Do you have a doctor who is a geriatric physician?
❖ Do you hide your feelings of despair?
❖ Do you try to do everything yourself because you think only you can best do the caretaking?
❖ Do you refuse help?
❖ Do you "put on a happy face" when you feel like you are sinking inside?
❖ Do you delegate tasks such as

grocery shopping, picking up medication, asking for help in feeding, outings, etc.?

If you answered yes to any of these questions, the Step Seven exercise may be helpful.

STEP SEVEN: EXERCISE

Make a list of the tasks that you could use help with (picking up medications, taking the person on an outing, playing cards, sharing a dessert, filling out forms, and taking your kids out for some fun, etc.). Next to the task, write the name of someone you know who would be able to help you.

Make a list of your fears in delegating.

Make a list of ways being compassionate is a gift for the person helping you.

Each day, call a friend.

Call the Alzheimer's Association and other support groups.

STEP SEVEN- BREATHING

Go back to the first exercise in breathing and try to do it again. It should seem second nature now that you've done it so many times. There is no specific exercise for step seven except to review the different step exercises and keep practicing the ones that work for you. Keep in mind that you may find different variations more useful depending on your situation.

STEP SEVEN: AFFIRMATIONS

"I allow others to practice compassion."

"It is in the giving that we all receive."

"I delegate."

"By allowing others to help, I am helping myself."

BENEFITS OF STEP SEVEN

Joining a support group is the beginning of your own healing. Calling people, talking with others who care about you, and even helping other caretakers helps to decrease your helplessness and enhances your connectedness. Being connected with other caregivers allows compassion to spread.

In a support group, you can express the normal feelings of guilt, sadness, anger, loneliness, and numbness. This allows you to process and let go of discomfort in your mind, body, and spirit. It allows you to practice acceptance, which is the key to your serenity. We cannot do it alone. It is the power of the whole that heals each of us as individuals and allows us to move on to the next indicated choice, often intuitively through the guidance of compassion and goodwill.

"Love is patient, love is kind. It does not envy, it does not boast, it is not proud. It is not rude, it is not self-seeking, it is not easily angered, it keeps no record of wrongs. Love does not delight in evil but rejoices with the truth. It always protects, always trusts, always hopes, always perseveres." – Anonymous

EPILOGUE: SAYING GOODBYE

Some call Alzheimer's "the long good-bye" and I leave you with a few closing thoughts.

Grief is a normal response to any loss, and the stages of loss are similar for many people. Join a support group to discuss feelings such as denial, anger, depression. When you are supported in the process of grieving, you can reach toward a final stage of acceptance more easily. All of these responses are normal and necessary along a path that is mentally and spiritually compassionate.

Your husband or wife or loved one may not be the person you "know" any more; the disease has changed him or her to someone you do not recognize. It is normal to feel deep grief about this loss.

Your life as you have known it is not the same; it is forever altered as a result of this disease. This is also a loss, and it is necessary to grieve.

You may be compassionate in choosing a facility that your loved one will be safer in and better suited to rather than being at home with you or living on her own.

You will look at suffering and death every day that you interact with a person with Alzheimer's because her mind is dying every day.

You may lose the image of who you thought the person was. Alzheimer's can open a Pandora's box of truths that may have been kept secret; as the disease progresses, the person's ability to "edit" their statements declines. She may begin to use profanity. She may act out repressed feelings and relate stories that she kept secret such as rape, combat events, fire, or deaths. This can be shocking to caretakers.

When presented with these "truths," there is sometimes no way to check what is reality. We only know that it is real to the person with Alzheimer's, and we can accept this with compassion and empathy.

Be generous in your care and loving to the person you are caring for and be equally generous and loving to yourself. It is in the giving we receive, and in the receiving that we give the endless circle of compassion and love.

To laugh is to risk appearing the fool.

To weep is to risk appearing sentimental.

To reach out for another is to risk involvement.

To expose feelings is to risk exposing your true self.

To place your ideas, your dreams, before a crowd is
to risk their loss.

To love is to risk not being loved in return.

To live is to risk dying.

To hope is to risk failure.

But risks must be taken.

Because the greatest hazard in life is to risk nothing.

If you risk nothing and do nothing, you dull your spirit.

You may avoid suffering and sorrow,

But you cannot learn, feel, change, grow, love, and live.

Chained by your attitude, you are a slave.

You have forfeited your freedom.

Only if you risk are you free.

— *Anonymous*

Closing Thoughts

Timelessness is being present, filling your heart with compassion.

Good will is contagious. We all mirror each other—families, facilities, corporations, communities, and other cultures.

We all need connection. It is communicated through acceptance, awareness, and contribution to a purpose that gives meaning to our lives.

Humor is a connecting force. It is the type of empathy that connects us immediately. Having the ability to laugh at yourself and with another person creates an instant moment of wordless bonding.

I hope that you will use the steps outlined here. Your mind and heart are already demonstrating your desire to be a compassionate caretaker.

I am grateful for you, dear reader, and for my connection with your good will to make the world a nurturing place of kindness, love, tolerance, and serenity. We cannot do it alone and I thank you for sharing my journey and I trust you will share yours with others. Your open heart is the door to infinite joy.

RESOURCES

Alzheimer's Disease Education and Referral (ADEAR) Center
P.O. Box 8250
Silver Spring, MD 20907-8250
(800) 438-4380
www.nia.nih.gov/Alzheimers

Alzheimer's Association
225 North Michigan Avenue, Suite 1700
Chicago, IL 60601-7633
(800) 272-3900
www.alz.org

Alzheimer's Foundation of America
322 8th Avenue, 7th Floor
New York, NY
(866) 232-8484
www.alzfdn.org

Children of Aging Parents
P.O. Box 167
Richboro, PA 18954-0167
(800) 227-7294
www.caps4caregivers.org

National Family Caregivers Association
10400 Connecticut Avenue, Suite 500
Kensington, MD 20895-3944
(800) 896-3650
www.thefamilycaregiver.org

National Hospice and Palliative Care Organization
1700 Diagonal Road, Suite 625
Alexandria, VA 22314
www.nhpco.org

Well Spouse Association
63 West Main Street, Suite H
Freehold, NJ 07728
www.wellspouse.org

For more information on Alzheimer's,
go to www.mariapertik.com.

CPSIA information can be obtained at www.ICGtesting.com
Printed in the USA
244581LV00001B/40/P